Collins

An Imprint of HarperCollinsPublishers

SEPHORA

THE BEAUTY AUTHORITY

the **ultimate guide** to
makeup, skin, and **hair**
from the beauty authority

by MELISSA SCHWEIGER

HarperCollins books may be purchased for educational, business, or sales promotional use. For information please write: Special Markets Department, HarperCollins Publishers, 10 East 53rd Street, New York, NY 10022.

FIRST EDITION

Designed by Lorie Pagnozzi and Bernadette Fitzpatrick

Library of Congress Cataloging-in-Publication Data

Schweiger, Melissa.
  Sephora: the ultimate guide to makeup, skin, and hair from the beauty authority/by Melissa Schweiger.—1st ed.
    p. cm.
ISBN 978-0-06-146640-3
1. Beauty, Personal. 2. Cosmetics. I. Sephora (Firm). II. Title.

RA776.98.S33 2007
646.7'2—dc22

2007050496

08 09 10 11 12   ID2 /RRD   10 9 8 7 6 5 4 3 2 1

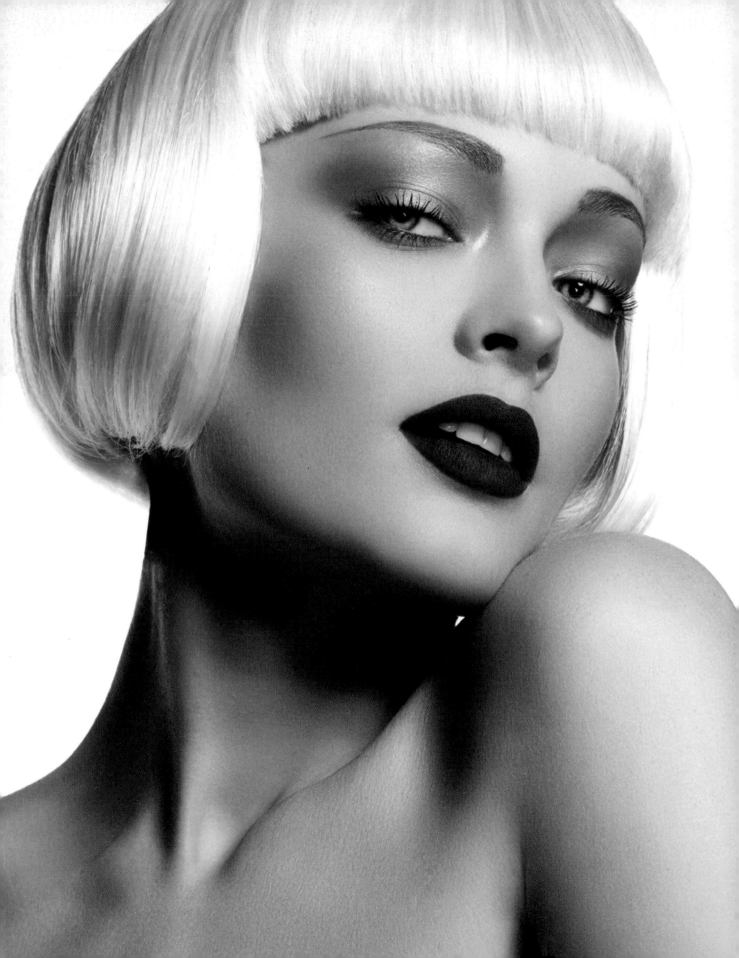

contents

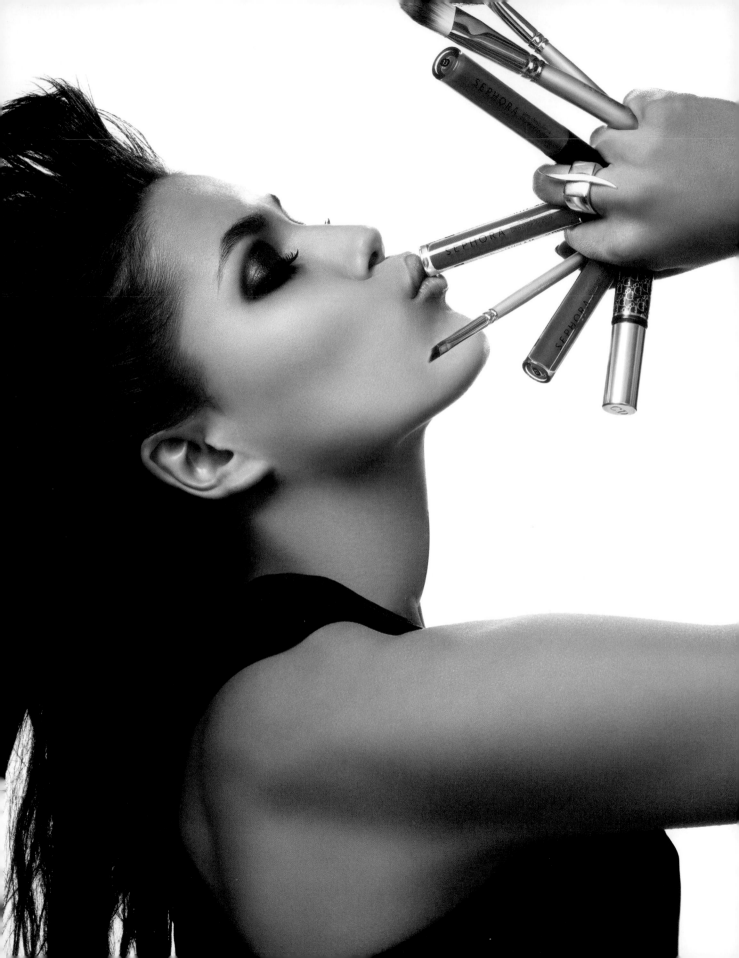

foreword

Since first setting foot in the United States in 1998, Sephora has become so much more than just a retailer. The palpable energy I feel every time I walk into one of our stores is truly contagious. Whether it's the most seasoned beauty addict, or someone taking her first dip into the world of cosmetics, never have I witnessed so many people so excited about beauty. That wild enthusiasm also holds true for the Sephora staff. The way we get giddy every time a new product lands on our desks, you'd think we'd never seen a lip gloss before. Our offices are a flurry of ideas, inspirations, and of course, beauty secrets. So we felt the time had come to divulge these amazing tips and tricks to you.

Over the past ten years, Sephora stores have been tempting women out of their comfort zones, and those were our exact intentions with this book. We've paired serious skin care, product, and ingredient education with inspiring ideas and easy-to-follow steps for amazing hair and makeup looks. You'll also find peppered throughout words of wisdom and top-secret beauty tips from the founders, skin care experts, and makeup artists that make Sephora truly the most beauty-full place on earth. Get ready to play, touch, feel, and try like a pro!

Enjoy!

Betsy Olum
Senior Vice President, Marketing
Sephora

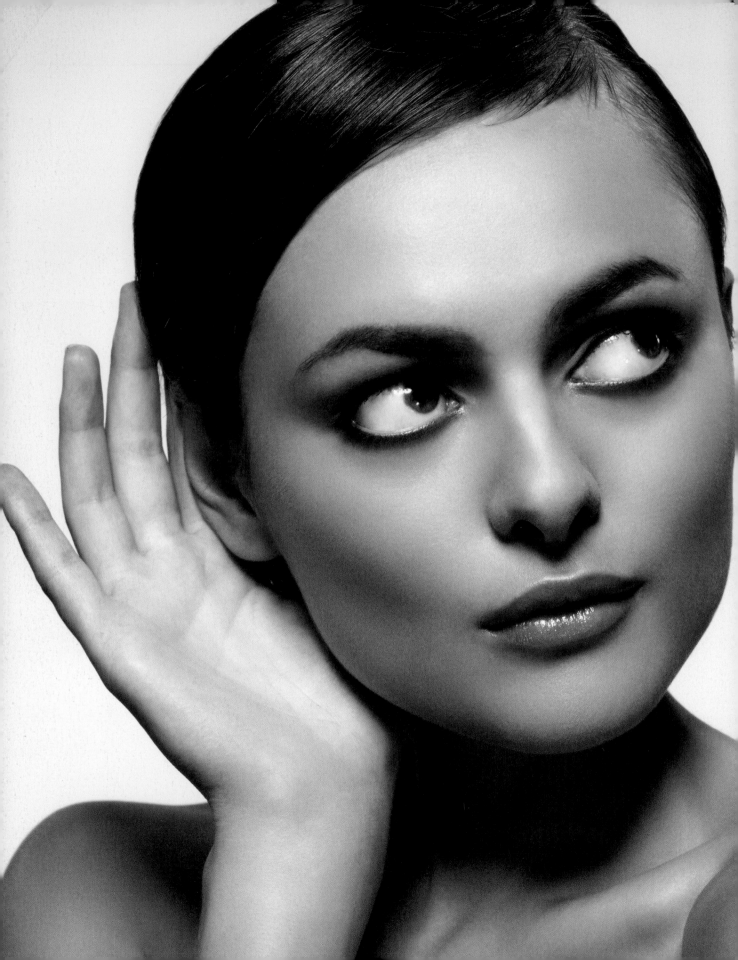

what is beauty?

We live in a world full of beauty. Sometimes it stares you directly in the face; other times, it's a little harder to find. But one thing is clear: Beauty means something different to everyone. Sephora's insiders each have their own unique, inspiring, and creative ways of defining beauty. Some of their ideas may even change *your* definition.

JERROD BLANDINO, founder of too faced: *"Beauty is confidence and a kick-ass style that's unique to you. It's about reinventing yourself throughout life. Don't stop at pretty——go for gorgeous all the time. Life isn't a dress rehearsal."*

Dr. Nicholas Perricone, founder of n.v. perricone m.d. cosmeceuticals: *"True beauty is radiant health. Aim for perfect health, and practice balance and moderation in everything you do. Follow the anti-inflammatory lifestyle and you can achieve optimal health and beauty. The interaction and synergy between diet and lifestyle, and our health, well-being, and longevity, holds the key to how well or how poorly we age."* .

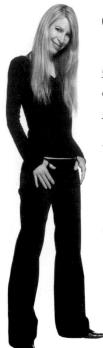

Carol Shaw, founder of lorac: *"You're as beautiful as you feel. Feeling beautiful in your own skin is true beauty, and that shines through. When you think you're beautiful, that's all that matters. It doesn't matter what anyone else thinks, says, does, or looks like. That's why makeup exists, to help women enhance their own beauty. Even just taking five minutes in the morning to put on a little blush and a little mascara will help you have a better day."*

Dr. Fredric Brandt, founder of dr. brandt skin care: *"Beauty is the best version of you that YOU can be. If you start comparing yourself to actresses or models, there's always going to be somebody who looks better than you. Besides, you don't even know what they really look like in real life! Just concentrate on having the healthiest skin that you can have."*

Karen Behnke, founder of juice beauty: *"Beauty is about being passionate in whatever you do—family, life, work. Passion makes people beautiful."*

Anthony Sosnick, founder of anthony logistics: *"Beauty means looking good and feeling good about yourself. One of the joys of being in this business is hearing 'thank you for making this product, it made me feel better about myself.' I think skin care is even better than clothing, because it's at your core."*

Lisa Price, founder of carol's daughter: *"Beauty is by nature. By that I mean that beauty is inherent in every single person. It's not something you can put on or take off."*

Sean "Diddy" Combs, founder of sean john: *"I believe beauty takes many shapes and forms. Beauty, to me, is confidence in who you are and what you believe in. When you're true to your own personal style, you can't help but exude a certain coolness and self-assurance. That's where true beauty lies: in the ability to be confident, to express your own individuality, and to strive to be the best you can be. Oh—and women, all women are beautiful!"*

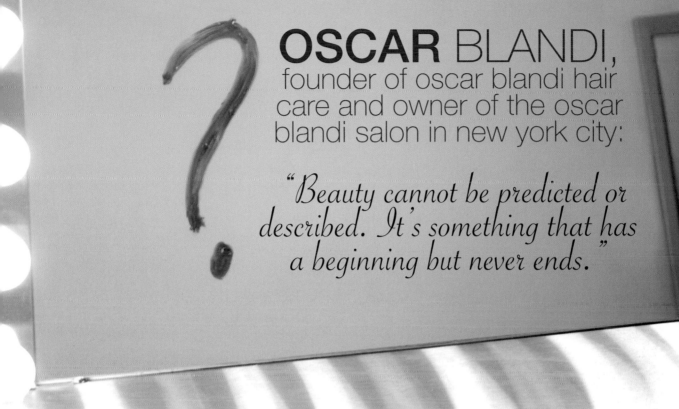

OSCAR BLANDI,
founder of oscar blandi hair care and owner of the oscar blandi salon in new york city:

"Beauty cannot be predicted or described. It's something that has a beginning but never ends."

Dr. Howard Murad, founder of murad: *"Someone who is immediately welcoming, someone who makes you feel comfortable—that's a beautiful person. You have to take a whole body approach to beauty. Many of my patients think that their skin is a separate organ, but it's not   it's connected by blood vessels to the heart, the liver, and the brain, so if any of those parts are damaged, then your skin will be damaged. That's why eating well, exercising, and wearing sunscreen are all so important."*

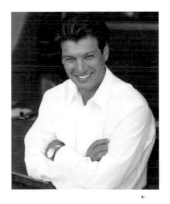

Frédéric Fekkai, owner of frédéric fekkai salons and founder of fekkai hair care: *"Chassez le naturel, il revient au galop! The English translation is: if you chase the natural, it will come back full gallop, meaning don't fight who you are or what you look like—just work with it."*

Hana Zalzal, founder of cargo cosmetics: *"Beauty is loving who you are, embracing the way you look, and continuing to make the most of both with a great haircut, neat brows, and some makeup basics. Makeup should be your servant, not your master. It should allow you to play, create, and evolve—it's a great tool for self-expression. Makeup is not permanent, so have fun with it!"*

Maureen Kelly, creator of tarte: *"Beauty comes in all sizes and ages—it's an attitude! It's more than just about looking like a model or a movie star. It's about feeling your best, believing in yourself, and having the emotion to translate through your facial expressions and body movements."*

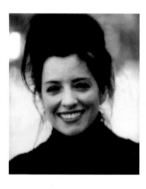

Cristina Carlino, founder of philosophy: *"Beauty is as beauty does. We're remembered not by what we looked like, but how we behaved and changed the lives of others."*

Dany Sanz, creator of make up for ever: *"Beauty can be bold or natural, but it always has to be in harmony with the individual."*

Wende Zomnir, creator of urban decay: *"Beauty is a true expression of who you are. The coolest girls I know are never the ones with the prettiest faces or the best bodies; they're the ones with their own unique style and look. They are the ones who are true to who they are."*

Jean Ford, cofounder of benefit: *"Beauty is a state of mind. What's beautiful to one person isn't necessarily to another. Beauty stops you in your tracks. Engages your eyes. Away from the ordinary, to the extraordinary."*

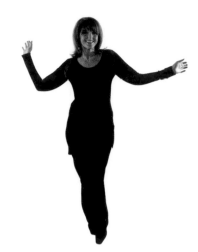

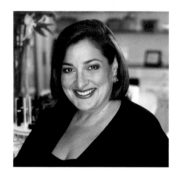

Laura Geller, founder of laura geller makeup: *"Beauty means to me that a woman should grow into herself every year. To stop fighting the law of gravity—it's our birthright to look and feel good about ourselves in a way that we can control. A sixty-year-old woman who has never gone under the knife, but is enhanced because she wears her makeup correctly, looks so much more beautiful than a woman who's been pulled, lifted, and injected."*

Ole Henriksen, founder of ole henriksen: *"Beauty means taking pride in caring for your appearance. Focus on eating deliciously healthy foods, take time to practice a fitness routine that energizes and strengthens your body, and don't forget to recharge your batteries and spend quality time with family and loved ones."*

Cristina Bartolucci, cofounder of duwop:

"There's a saying that truth is beauty, beauty is truth. When a woman is really comfortable in her own skin, it shines through with or without makeup."

Sue Devitt of sue devitt studio cosmetics: *"Beauty starts internally. You have to eat healthfully, do yoga to stretch your body, Pilates to strengthen your core, and cardio to burn fat. Another important factor is to make time for yourself—choose some healthy things that make you feel great and do them for yourself."*

Victoria Jackson, makeup artist: *"My mom always used to say 'Just wash your face, put on a little makeup, and go out there.' I grew up in a family where there was no money and I had to go out there and make my way. That was my mom's way of telling me not to let anything stop me. I learned that it's all about feeling and looking better. It's what I call the power of mascara. Just do your makeup and go out and conquer the world!"*

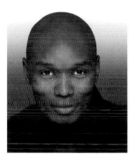

Ross Burton, national artistic director of lancôme:
"Beauty equals confidence. You can be the prettiest woman on the planet, but if you're not confident, it's not going to matter what reflection you see in the mirror."

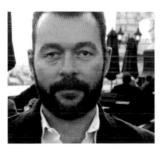

Dick Page, artistic director of shiseido:
"Makeup is a really good form of self-expression—it's your window into the world, it's how you first present yourself, and how people see you. Makeup is also the easiest and most accessible way to deal with fashion. Not many people can afford the handbags or the shoes, but everyone can afford lipstick."

Leslie Blodgett, ceo of bare escentuals: *"No matter what a woman looks like, the ones who have their chins up and a step that's a little bit faster—those are the people who define beauty for me. I meet women of all ages and the ones who have accepted themselves for who they are and what they look like are the most beautiful. They're perkier and happier. I feel the most beautiful when I start accepting what's happening to me as I get older and stop blaming myself. I know I'm starting to lose my neck and I can't prevent it from happening. Instead of getting depressed about it, I just look at it and say 'Oh look, I'm getting another chin—that's kind of cute.' I have to look at it this way, because I'm not about to get a face-lift."*

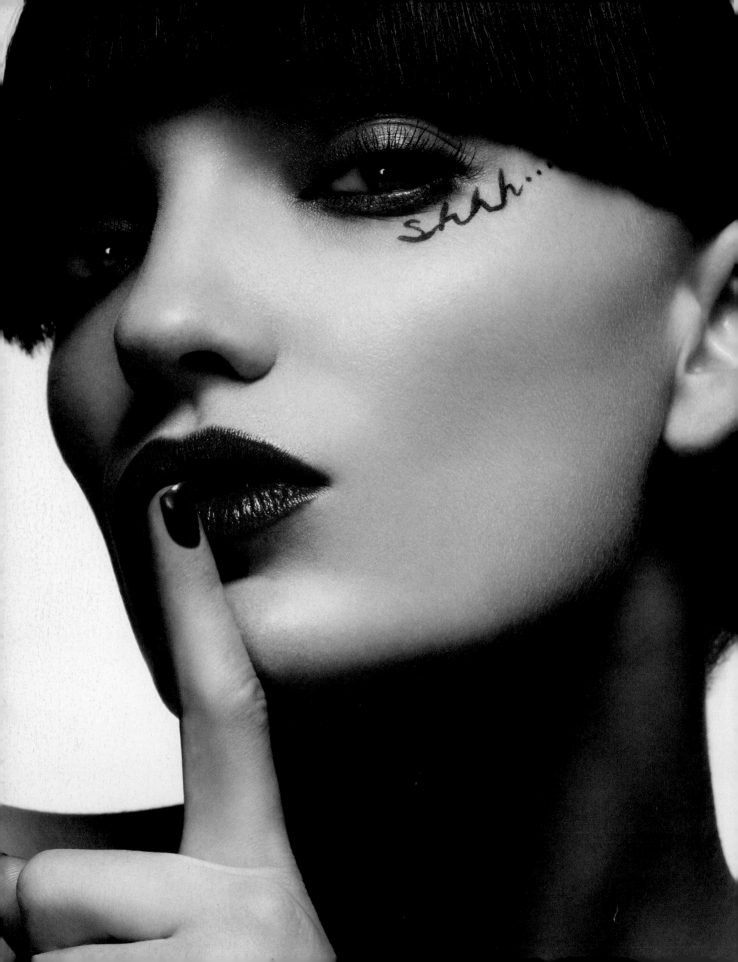

faking it

There's no harm in faking it once in a while, especially if it makes you look—
and feel—a little better. We're not suggesting doing something outrageously
artificial. Our version of going faux is subtle, sophisticated, sexy, and *tres* natural.
Playing up your already gorgeous features is a great place to start. "Enhance and
build your strengths and downplay your weaknesses," says makeup artist Victoria
Jackson. But when you're craving a touch more than what you've already got
(voluptuous lips, anyone?), then pay heed to the beauty secrets in this chapter. We
promise not to tell . . .

tip

"Apply body bronzer to your legs before you apply your makeup so it has time to set and dry while you're doing your face."

—Carol Shaw

FAKE . . . LONG, LUSCIOUS LEGS

We're going to let you in on a little secret. Supermodels have cellulite. We swear it's true. Anyone who's ever sat front row during fashion week will attest to this glorious news. But that doesn't mean we all still don't dream of owning a pair of long, lean, and perfectly smooth stems. Get a leg up with these tricks and tips and we bet you'll be hot to trot—that is, unless you plan on sashaying down a harshly lit runway in hot pants the size of a postage stamp.

smooth operator

Orange peel, cottage cheese . . . whatever culinary pseudonym you've decided to bestow on those lovely lumps on your thighs, we all know its proper name—cellulite. There is some good news and some bad news when it comes to fighting the c-word. "Tackling cellulite is a multifold process," says Ann Marie Cilmi, director of development and education at Bliss Spas. "It has to be addressed through diet (eight bags of cookies a day does not a cellulite-free thigh make), via stimulation of circulation (our thin-thighed ancestors were not known to sit in ergonomically correct office chairs for ten hours a day), and exercise (nobody walks twenty-six miles to get fresh water anymore . . . it may be saving us time, but it's not saving our thighs!)."

Diet is indeed critical to wiping out cellulite. "To encourage healthy, hydrated cells and connective tissue, I recommend foods such as soy or tofu, cauliflower, spinach, oranges, and tomatoes. They all have lecithin, which strengthens skin and makes it harder for cellulite to show through," says Dr. Howard Murad. He also suggests loading up on things like pistachio nuts, walnuts, pomegranates, goji berries, broccoli, and green tea. "Feeding the skin is equally as important as applying topical products. When you use topical products, you address approximately 20 percent of the skin, the epidermis. The remaining 80 percent, the dermis, requires nourishment from foods and dietary supplements. Foods rich in essential fatty acids, antioxidants, lecithin, glucosamine, and amino acids encourage healthy, strong blood vessels and connective tissue," he says. "Cellulite, for example, is a direct result of poor circulation caused by weakened blood vessels and connective tissue that has deteriorated. By feeding the body the key elements for healthy collagen and elastin production, you can reduce the appearance of cellulite and skin that has lost its firmness."

brush out cellulite

To stimulate the movement of toxins through the body so that they don't pool under the skin and lead to the appearance of cellulite, increase your surface circulation with Bliss's dry-brushing technique, to be done on a daily basis:

1 With a clean, firm, natural-bristle brush, begin brushing at your feet upward toward your heart, using enough pressure to stimulate circulation, but not enough to bruise you.

2 Brush in circles around your knees and at the top and inner areas of your thighs.

3 Circle your brush around your abdominal wall, in the direction of your intestines (from the lower right side, move up and across above your belly button, then down the left side).

rub out cellulite

Modern technology has brought us many useful things: cell phones, the Internet, and high-tech anticellulite creams! Here, our favorites.

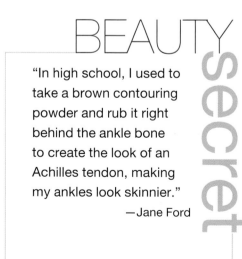

BEAUTY secret

"In high school, I used to take a brown contouring powder and rub it right behind the ankle bone to create the look of an Achilles tendon, making my ankles look skinnier."

—Jane Ford

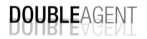

DOUBLEAGENT

"I use Carol's Daughter Peppermint Foot Oil all over my legs—and on my entire body—to cool me off on a hot day."

—Lisa Price

MURAD THE CELLULITE SOLUTION

Dr. Murad has created a trio of products that, according to clinical studies, reduce the appearance of cellulite by up to 69 percent and improve the overall appearance of skin by up to 80 percent. These revolutionary formulas, packed with vitamins, antioxidants, and humectants, are designed to stimulate circulation

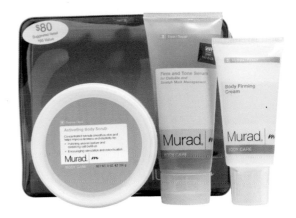

while polishing and firming to reveal tighter, smoother, more hydrated skin. The Cellulite Solution includes Murad Activating Body Scrub (a concentrated formula that smoothes the skin as it firms and helps improve elasticity), Murad Firm and Tone Serum (improves the overall appearance of skin and reduces the appearance of cellulite), and Murad Body Firming Cream (a patented, ultrarich body cream that helps keep skin young and supple).

CLARINS BODY SHAPING SUPPLEMENT

Transform any body cream into a cellulite-eradicating work of wonder with just a few drops of Body Shaping Supplement. Formulated with seven key botanicals with proven refining and streamlining properties, including *Baccharis* (an exclusive aromatic plant found in the Amazon that helps inhibit the development of fat tissue), *Hortonia* (a small shrub from Sri Lanka that helps block the formation of new adipocytes—aka fat cells), *Cangzhu, Agrimony* (a plant found in Africa, Europe, and Asia that enhances the elimination of water and toxins), and caffeine to help increase circulation and lymphatic drainage.

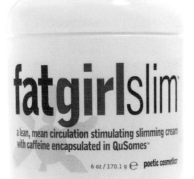

BLISS FAT GIRL SLIM
For firmer skin that looks less sponge-like, turn to this fat-hating treatment. "This advanced technology adipose antagonist (which in layman's terms means it visibly diminishes those dastardly dimples) features QuSome-encapsulated caffeine molecules for quick and targeted delivery of the skin-slimming stuff of choice of supermodels and spokespeople," says Bliss's Cilmi.

picks

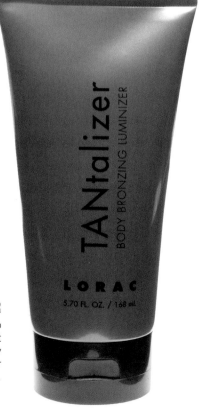

BENEFIT BATHINA BODY SO FINE

This ultraluminescent body balm with a soft sheen will make your legs look as though they're sheathed in silk stockings. Famous TV stars love Bathina because it creates the appearance of flawless limbs on camera.

LORAC TANTALIZER

"This will instantly turn your legs into supermodel legs. It gives you that warm, golden tan look—it's totally transforming," says LORAC founder Carol Shaw.

MICHAEL KORS LEG SHINE

Glide this bronze-tinted shimmer stick along legs, knees, and ankles for a sleek, sexy look that will make bare legs look healthy and glowing—and smelling gorgeous (it's infused with the tuberose Michael scent).

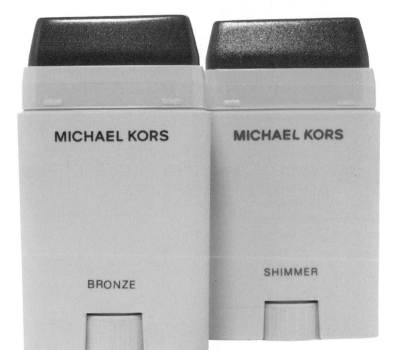

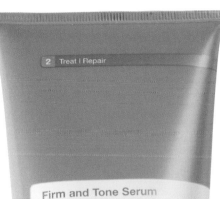

MURAD FIRMING BRONZER SPF 15 FOR FACE & BODY

This face and body bronzer beautifies with triple action benefits. Broad-spectrum SPF 15 protection blocks damaging UV rays, temporarily increasing skin firmness by 32 percent in just fifteen minutes. The believable bronze washes off easily with soap and water.

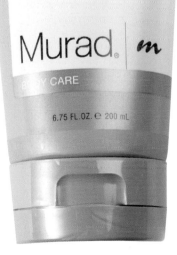

NARS BODY GLOW

Douse your body in this cult-favorite transparent chocolate-shimmer body oil. Monoi de Tahiti oil, a natural skin elixir, gives the skin a buttery-soft, healthy gleam.

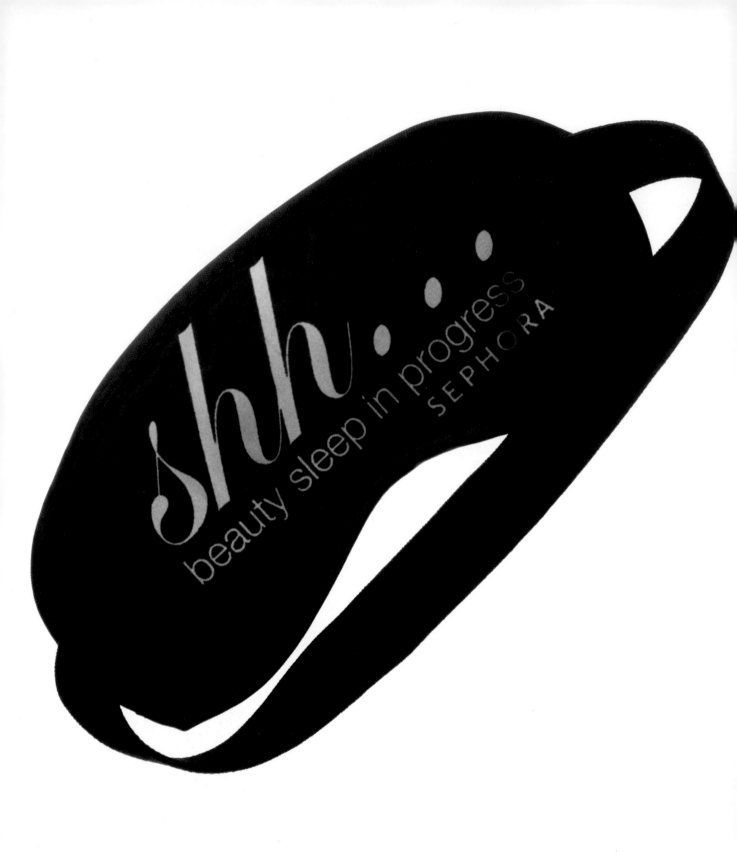

FAKE . . . EIGHT HOURS OF AMAZING SLEEP

You look tired. Next to "You have a huge pimple," there's no other phrase in the English language that makes you want to run for cover more. Exhaustion, like parking tickets, is an unfortunate side effect of everyday living. But that doesn't mean you have to look it. Whether your night consisted of hours of restless tossing and turning, cramming to meet a deadline, or some other late-night dalliance, the effect on your complexion is still the same. Hello, puffy! Hi there, sallow! What's up, dark circles? Trick your public—and yourself—into thinking you had a seamless eight hours of REM sleep.

eye-openers

Wearing too much eye makeup when you're tired is like sporting a snug half-shirt the day after Thanksgiving. It only points a big, red arrow directly to the problem area. But *not* wearing anything around the eyes can be just as jarring. It's all about subtle little tricks.

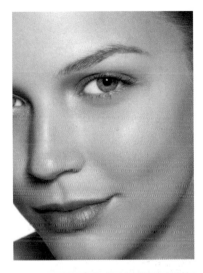

- "Use hints of gold shadow around the eye," says DuWop's Cristina Bartolucci. "Apply a tiny bit of intense gold shadow at the inner corners of your eye and then wash it over your lids."

- "My little trick is to use a flesh-colored eyeliner on the inside of the lid; this opens the eye and blends into the skin tone, killing any pink or redness the inner lid may have," says Shane Paish, global makeup advisor for Dior.

- An eyelash curler and a couple coats of mascara can do more to wake you up than a double espresso. "Get the curler as close as possible to the lashline without pinching the skin," says makeup artist Dick Page. "The key is to stop as soon as you feel it bump against the lid." Page also suggests using several pulsing squeezes down the lash until you get to the tips.

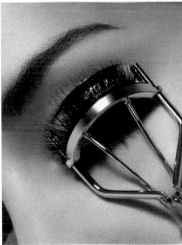

tip

To avoid dark circles and under-eye bags, try sleeping with extra pillows. Gravity helps fight the accumulation of fluid under the eyes.

dark circles, dark schmircles!

"Dark circles are every woman's nemesis," says Laura Geller, makeup artist and founder of Laura Geller Makeup. Indeed, it's not just lack of sleep that will cause these extra-special shadows to appear. We can also thank our great-grandmothers (dark circles can be genetic), allergies, eating gobs of soy sauce–laden sushi (fluid retention is a dark-circle culprit), and aging, which causes the skin around the eyes to thin, allowing veins to show. "If you're just trying to cover a little darkness, bring your foundation right up under your eyes and then gauge how much concealer you need. If you can still see shadows, it's time to bring in heavier artillery," says Geller. Eliminate the enemy with these dark circle–erasing steps.

1. Locate the problem

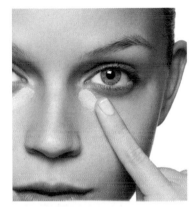

Dark circles rarely form all the way underneath the eyes. If you're sending them a cease and desist, you have to find them first. "Look straight into the mirror and then slowly tilt your chin down and suddenly the circles will pop out—it's actually kind of scary," says DuWop's Cristina Bartolucci. The dark circles in question are those half-moons of blueness beginning right above the tear duct, close to the nose.

2. Conceal

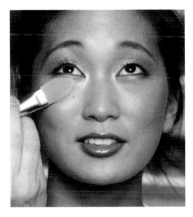

"The pinky finger is nature's little dark circle–concealing tool," says Bartolucci. "It fits perfectly in that half-moon area." Dab a peachy-toned concealer, to counteract the blue-green circle, onto the side of your pinky and tap it right into the dark area. "Don't extend the concealer into the temple area—it will only accentuate any fine lines or wrinkles," says Sue Devitt. "The only thing you should be using in that area are eye-treatment products or foundation."

check your bags

"Concealer's not going to do anything when it comes to under-eye bags," says Dick Page, artistic director for Shiseido The Makeup. "So I'll use a dot of really vivid pearl highlighter on the inner corner of the eye, under the lower lids, and on the outer corner of the brow." The highlighter acts as an optical illusion, catching the light and making the eyes appear more awake. "It's similar to what actresses used to do in the theater," explains Page. "They would apply a dot of red in the corners of the eyes, because from a distance it gave the impression of brightness."

in the pink

"You tend to lose color on the face when you haven't slept, so the cheeks need brightening," says Victoria Jackson. A baby-pink blush works wonders for waking up an exhausted complexion. But be sure to blend! "You should never see where blush begins or ends," says Lancôme's Ross Burton. "It should look flushed, not applied." To get that healthy I-spent-the-last-week-reading-a-romance-novel-in-a-hammock-on-St. Croix look, Burton suggests using a creamy-textured blush on the apples of the cheeks and then blending with a foundation brush.

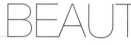

BEAUTY secrets

"Deflect attention away from the eye area with a bright lipstick."

—Jane Ford

"When you wake up in the morning, fill your sink with a combination of cold water and ice cubes. Dip a terrycloth washcloth into the sink, wring it out, and then press it across your face five to ten times. Your complexion will truly be revived and awakened."

—Ole Henriksen

"Chewing really strong mint gum wakes me up if I'm tired."

—Cristina Bartolucci

pick
picks

faking it:
good night's sleep

TOO FACED WRINKLE INJECTION

Watch your wrinkles and fine lines pull a disappearing act! Laugh lines, deep crevices, and forehead furrows are instantly obliterated, thanks to the crease-relief formula in this magic tube.

AMAZING COSMETICS AMAZING CONCEALER

This superconcentrated concealer is for those times you want to wear a paper bag over your head. Its professional formula completely covers dark circles, age spots, and blemishes without a hint that anything unsightly is lurking underneath.

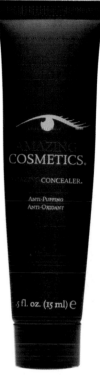

LORAC UNDERCOVER LOVER

Made specifically for the under-eye area, this breakthrough concealer is packed with nourishing antioxidants and light-reflecting ingredients that shave ten years off your face. Apply after foundation.

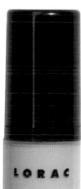

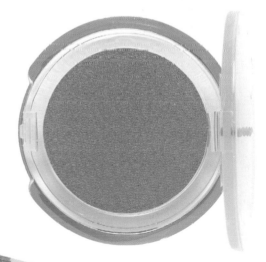

BENEFIT EYE BRIGHT

"We call this a nap-in-a-stick!" says Benefit cofounder Jane Ford. "It brightens the entire area around the eyes and makes you look wide awake."

SEPHORA BLUSH IN RUSTIC ROSE

Brighten up your entire face in just one sweep with this soft, blendable, pretty rosy-pink shade. Cheeks will look naturally flushed and full of radiance.

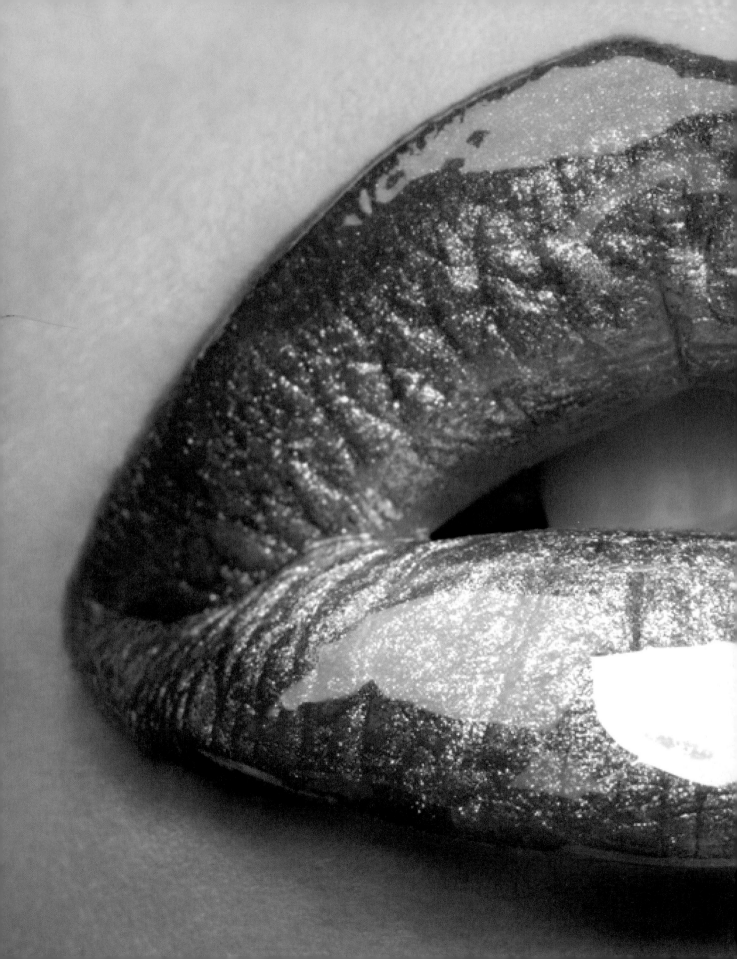

FAKE .... A SEXY, JUICY POUT

"A full pout is a sign of youth and a hallmark of beauty," says Randi Shinder, founder of Fusion Beauty. "The mouth is incredibly provocative," agrees Benefit cofounder Jane Ford. Thankfully, painfully expensive injections aren't the only way to achieve pillow lips. Modern technology, along with a few key makeup tricks, will have your lips on the fat track faster than you can say "kiss me."

BEAUTY
tip

Toss pout plumpers
after one year, which
is about when their
super lip-enlarging
powers begin to
diminish.

plump up the volume!

How to get ginormous lips in five easy steps from celebrity makeup artist and DuWop cofounder Cristina Bartolucci:

1 Apply a coat of Fresh Sugar Lip Balm to lips, then wipe off after thirty seconds with a warm washcloth. This will exfoliate and condition the lips at the same time.

2 Slather DuWop Lip Venom all over the lips. Wait ten minutes and wipe off.

3 The edges of the lip are now superprominent and easy to line, thanks to the swelling effects of Lip Venom. With a nude lip liner, cover the entire lip and buff it sheer with your fingers. "Then you're going to push the envelope," says Bartolucci. "Go right to the edge of that newly exaggerated lip line with the nude pencil and smudge it with your fingertip, just over the edge."

4 Layer! "The secret to beautiful lips is layering sheer over sheer," says Bartolucci. First start with a lip stain, then either do a sheer-formulated lipstick or a tinted gloss.

5 Dot a shimmery pink, gold, or silver gloss onto the center of the lower lip.

beauty History

In 1999, Lip Venom launches and becomes the beauty industry's first lip plumper . . . by accident! The original idea was to create a product that gave lips the sexy, flushed color that came after hours of kissing. But what they got instead was a spicy blend of essential oils that produced ultra-augmented lips.

makeup artist technique: lip liner

Contouring the lips with lip liner gives dimension to the lips and a sophisticated definition to the entire mouth, but it takes skill. Here, makeup artist Vincent Longo on how to get that sharp, chic, and subtle contour:

BEAUTY tips

"A great way to find your perfect lip shade is by looking at the inside of your cheek and find a color that's two shades darker. That color is the most natural match for your lips."

—Jean Ford

"Dab a luminizer on the cupid's bow of the mouth and lips will look instantly plumper."

—Jerrod Blandino

1 With a sharply pointed neutral-hued lip liner, create a nice even shape on the bow of the lips. Then go to the left outer corner on the upper lip and trace the lip line with the liner back to the bow and repeat on the right side.

2 On the lower lip, trace the lip line starting from the outer left corner, going inward. Repeat on the other side. With a third stroke, combine the lines. Use a lip brush to smudge the line so it's not too harsh.

pretty smart

All lip plumpers are not created equal. Be sure to try before you buy, as some potions are much stronger than others and can cause major irritation to the lips and entire mouth area—not so sexy.

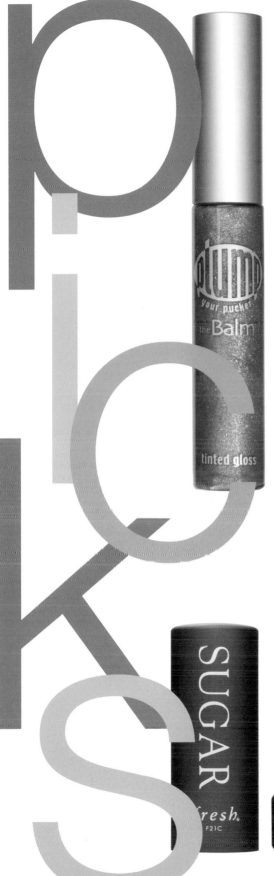

pi¢ks

faking it:
juicy lips

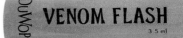

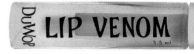

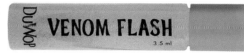

THEBALM LIP PLUMPER TINTED LIP GLOSS IN STRAWBERRY MY SHORTCAKE

To get maximum plumpness, add a touch of light, pink shimmer with this sweet-scented gloss to the center of your bottom lip.

DUWOP LIP VENOM

In a word: addictive! This cinnamon and ginger-infused gloss increases the circulation of the lips, leaving them deliciously plump and with a seductive, just-kissed color.

FUSION BEAUTY FULL OUT POUT SET

For natural-looking, fuller lips, turn to this treatment gloss and revolutionary lip liner that shapes, defines, and plumps lips.

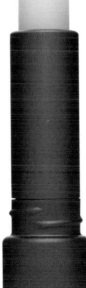

FRESH SUGAR LIP TREATMENT

Start any lip-plumping regimen with this must-own treatment. Essential fatty acids cushion the lips, while antioxidant grapeseed polyphenols and vitamins A, C, and E provide extra protection.

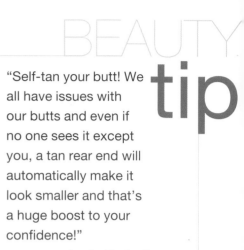

"Self-tan your butt! We all have issues with our butts and even if no one sees it except you, a tan rear end will automatically make it look smaller and that's a huge boost to your confidence!"

—Leslie Blodgett

FAKE . . . A GORGEOUS GOLDEN GLOW

When Coco Chanel stepped off a yacht after a Mediterranean holiday in the 1920s with a deep brown tone to her skin, the suntan look officially became fashionable, and our love-hate relationship with the sun was born. We heart a gorgeous, sienna hue, but do we love the inevitable wrinkle party and potential health problems that will happen down the road? Not so much. These staggering stats should have you running for the fake stuff: More than 95 percent of skin cancer is from exposure to the sun; 1.5 million new cases of skin cancer are diagnosed every day. There are nearly 8,000 melanoma deaths a year—that is one person every hour. So what's a tanorexic to do? Enter bronzers. "When we're feeling tired or sick, a good bronzer can really make you feel like you went on holiday for a week," says makeup artist Laura Geller. Smart, sophisticated, and—with the right direction—easy to use, bronzers and self-tanners have indeed become seasonless beauty essentials.

fool's gold

The right bronzer can transform you into a St. Tropez goddess with just a few flicks of the wrist, but to successfully snag a golden glow that's both flattering and convincing, you must select a shade that warms your complexion, rather than changes it. The goal is to appear gently kissed by the sun—not burnished like a bronzed statuette.

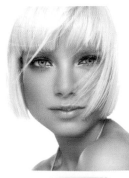

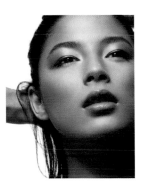

LIGHT COMPLEXIONS: Stick to sheer, cool bronzers that have a beige undertone. Anything too brown will be obvious and make your skin appear muddy.

MEDIUM COMPLEXIONS: Lucky ladies! You can pretty much get away with any bronzer, but your best bet will be one that's gold or brown (those hues really warm up your skin).

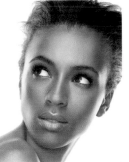

DARK COMPLEXIONS: Golden and brown-based bronzers look the most natural on you. If your skin is very dark, opt for a bronzer with more red or copper in it, which will really pop and give you a gorgeous, sunny color.

here comes the sun!

Application is everything when it comes to going faux. For the most realistic results, use a large fluffy brush and follow these steps:

1 Give your face a light dusting with a loose translucent powder before applying bronzer to matte any oils from the skin. If you apply color over skin that has moisture on it, the color will grab on to those oil slicks and it won't blend properly.

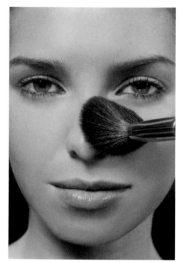

2 "Apply bronzer in the 'W' area on the face (the cheeks and the bridge of the nose), which is where the sun naturally hits," says Too Faced creator Jerrod Blandino. Give cheeks a light dusting first, then, in a circular motion, move the brush across the bridge of the nose without redipping the brush into the bronzer. "Using what's left on your brush, go into the hairline—it gives a great sculpt to the face and makes you look like you lost ten pounds," says Blandino.

3 Don't forget to sweep the bronzer onto your ears. "Bronzer is an illusion, and if your ears don't match the tan color of your complexion, the illusion is broken," says DuWop's Cristina Bartolucci.

4 "Every natural tan has a bit of burn underneath," says Blandino. To get a believable-looking tan with pink undertones and to counteract any muddiness, apply a bright-pink blush onto the apples of the cheeks.

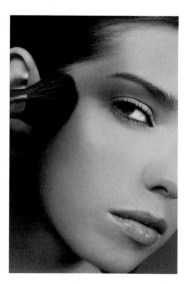

5 Don't neglect your neck—a glowing face and a pasty white neck is a beauty train wreck. "Use the residue on the brush left over from applying bronzer and dust it down your décolletage. To prevent creasing on the neck, keep your chin up when applying bronzer," says Benefit's Jane Ford.

put it
where? Apply
liquid bronzer to your lips atop clear lip gloss. The
result? A pout that's shimmery, sexy, yet oh-so-subtle.

golden glow FAQs

Q: What makeup colors look great against bronzed skin?

a: Choose colors that will pop against a tan backdrop. "Violet mascara, cool pinks around the eye, and a violet finish on the lips look amazing with bronze skin," says makeup artist Dick Page.

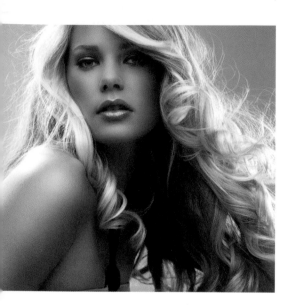

Q: How can I create sexy beach hair to go with my bronzed and beautiful new look?

a: "Braid your hair while it's still damp," advises Oscar Blandi. After towel-drying hair, create about five to ten braids of different sizes all over the head. "The key is to make sure the braids are imperfect, otherwise hair will look crimped instead of tousled," says Blandi. Curl the braids with a curling iron for major beach waves, or go over them with a flatiron for a smoother look. After hair is dry, take out the braids and use your fingers to give the hair a good shake.

Q: I want my hair to look naturally sun-kissed too! What do I do?

a: "Ask your colorist for a few strategically placed highlights," says Kyle White, senior colorist at the Oscar Blandi Salon. The thickest and brightest pieces should frame the face and regress in size and tone toward the crown—and always leave the depth underneath. "There's nothing more artificial-looking than heavy highlights woven way down at the nape of the neck," says White. "This would never happen naturally; the sun is exposed only to the top layer of hair."

beauty school: self-tanning

How to get a faux all-over glow, without making any faux pas:

1 Start in the shower. Shave your legs and use a loofah to slough off dead skin. Avoid using an exfoliator loaded with essential oils, as it may react with the self-tanner and cause splotchy, streaky areas.

2 Pat yourself dry post-shower. Put on a pair of disposable latex gloves and apply the tanner. Start by using a quarter-sized amount for each leg. Rub, rub, rub until you can't see even a trace of self-tanner. Now do the same for arms and chest. Pay extra-special attention to knees and elbows, where dry skin can catch the self-tanner.

3 Wash your hands. Apply a nickel-sized amount to backs of the hands and rub only the backs together.

4 Wait ten minutes before getting dressed. Stand in front of a fan to speed up the drying process.

sculpting tricks

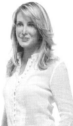

Randi Shinder, founder of Fusion Beauty's GlowFusion and self-professed faux tanning addict, uses her Air Glow Gun to create a six-pack, contour her arms, and enhance her décolletage. Here's how she does it:

BEAUTY tip

"After makeup application, use a light dusting of bronzer instead of translucent powder—it will set your makeup and give you a healthy glow."
—Cristina Bartolucci

- Obliques: "Contour the area where you would normally see definition in your abs by spraying the gun a few seconds longer on the area the lines of a six-pack would exist."

- Cleavage: "Outline and enhance the tops of the breasts by spraying the gun a teeny bit longer on the area where the top of the bra would hit."

- Arms: "Define your biceps or contour the triceps by spraying a bit longer directly onto the muscle."

treasure chest

In the quest for a perfect tan, don't forget to match your face to your cleavage! The faux glow on your face will disappear much faster than the bronze on your body, so finding a balance between the two—especially if you're wearing a low-cut top—is essential. "If the face is paler than the body, try and find a point between the two," says Dick Page. "Warm up the face a bit with a light wash of bronzer and blend with a foundation or blush brush very lightly, making sure there's no demarcation line around the neck and jaw." Page also suggests highlighting the clavicle and the tops of breasts if you're wearing a low-cut dress. "I tell brides all the time to be really aware of the tonalities of the face and body. You don't want to look as though you have a floating head in photographs."

faking it:
a golden glow

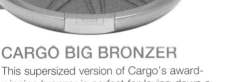

CARGO BIG BRONZER

This supersized version of Cargo's award-winning bronzer is perfect for laying down a wash of golden color anywhere! Sweep onto cheeks, décolletage—even arms and legs.

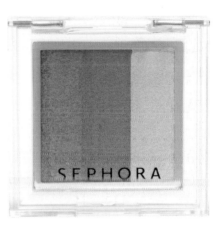

NARS THE MULTIPLE IN PALM BEACH

For the richest-looking tan around, dab this multitasking, cream-to-powder stick anywhere you see fit. Use your fingers to enhance and sculpt cheekbones, eyes, and the jawline.

GUERLAIN TERRACOTTA SPRAY SPF 10 BRONZING POWDER MIST

Deliver a streak-free Caribbean glow to hard-to-reach spots with this revolutionary bronzing mist. Bonus: Use it to contour by concentrating the mist a little bit longer on those areas you want to get noticed.

SEPHORA LUMINOUS TRIO IN BRONZE

This highlighting trio of shimmering shades of bronze leaves a twinkling veil of luminosity on face and body. Mix all three colors together or use them separately.

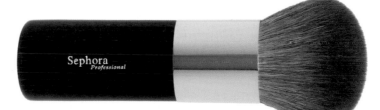

SEPHORA BRAND PROFESSIONEL PLATINUM BRONZER BRUSH

If you're going to use bronzer—and you want it to look realistic—you better have this tool in your kit. The strategically placed hairs have an uncanny way of getting bronzer in exactly the spots the sun would hit.

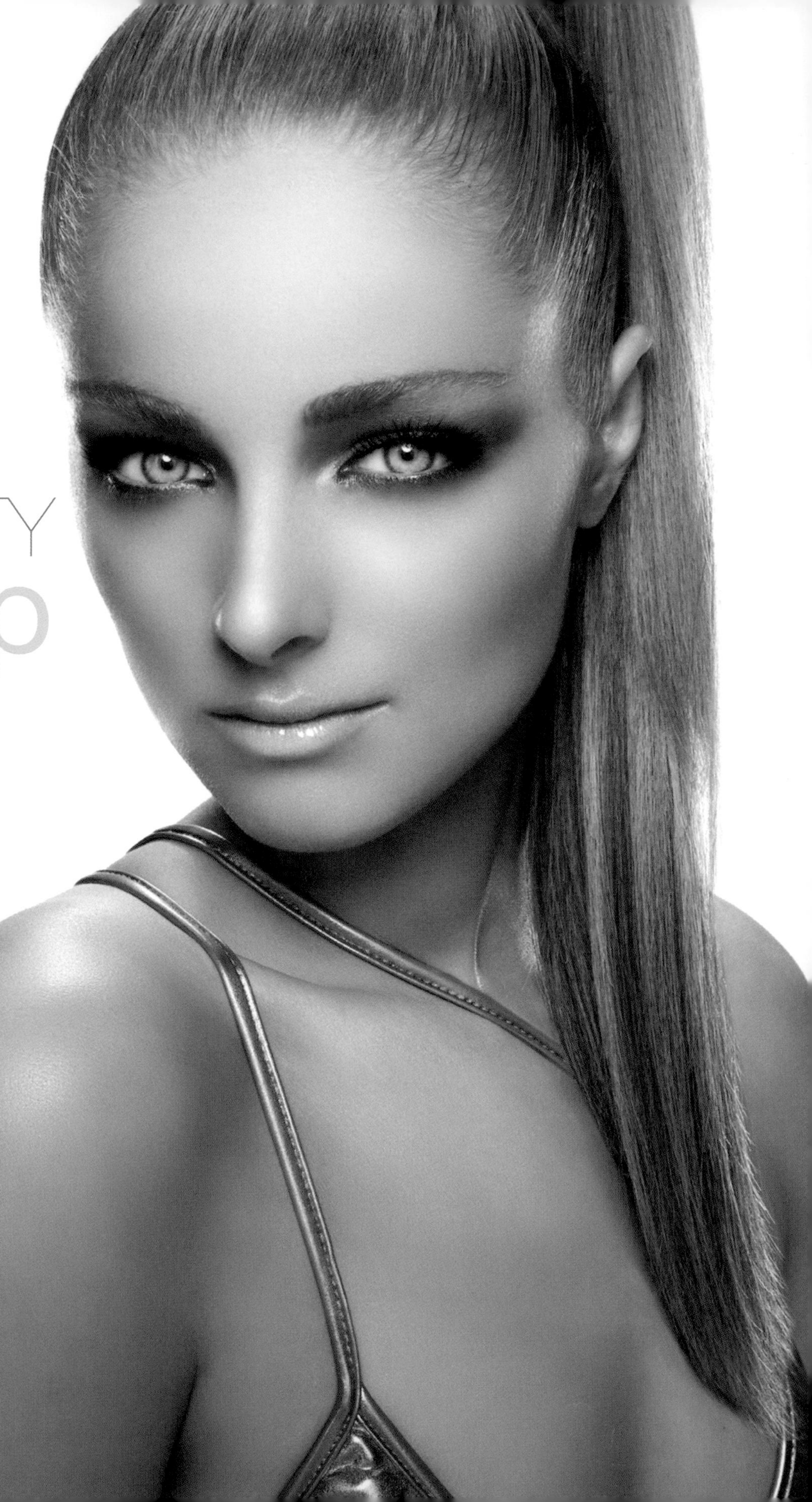

BEAUTY tip

Mix liquid bronzer with your foundation for an all-over glow.

Gently tap off your makeup brush before applying bronzer to shake off excess color.

FAKE . . . HIGH CHEEKBONES

High cheekbones are the beauty equivalent of a four-carat diamond ring. Every woman secretly covets one, even if she pretends she's happy with what she's got. Good news! Even if the genetic lottery didn't reward you with a pair of glamorously jutting cheekbones, you can still be the proud owner of a pair. As for the diamond ring, well, they're doing incredible things with cubic zirconia these days . . .

très cheek

Prominent cheekbones in four easy steps:

1 "Lightness brings out and darkness draws in," says celebrity makeup artist and LORAC founder Carol Shaw. "So you want to apply something light to the tops of your cheekbones to create the illusion of them being higher." On top of any foundation, dab a luminizing liquid on the high cheekbone area, so the light will reflect off that area and lift it up.

2 "Apply a baby-pink blush high as you can on the apple of your cheek, right underneath the iris of your eye underneath your bottom lashes," says makeup artist Sue Devitt. "This really lifts your cheeks and gives your entire face a youthful glow."

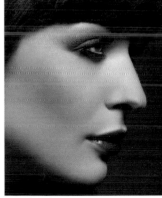

3 Since dark colors recess where they've been applied, you want to contour the hollows of the cheek with a darker color. Suck in your cheeks and sweep a taupe powder blush or a bronzer a couple shades darker than your skin tone into the hollows of the cheeks. The contour line should end below the apples of the cheeks. And blend! "You want to have all the colors working together, not three separate stripes," says Shaw.

4 "Gently use the color left on the brush and sweep it across the eyelids," says makeup artist Laura Geller. "It gives a really beautiful finish and it brings all the attention upward, making your cheekbones look even higher."

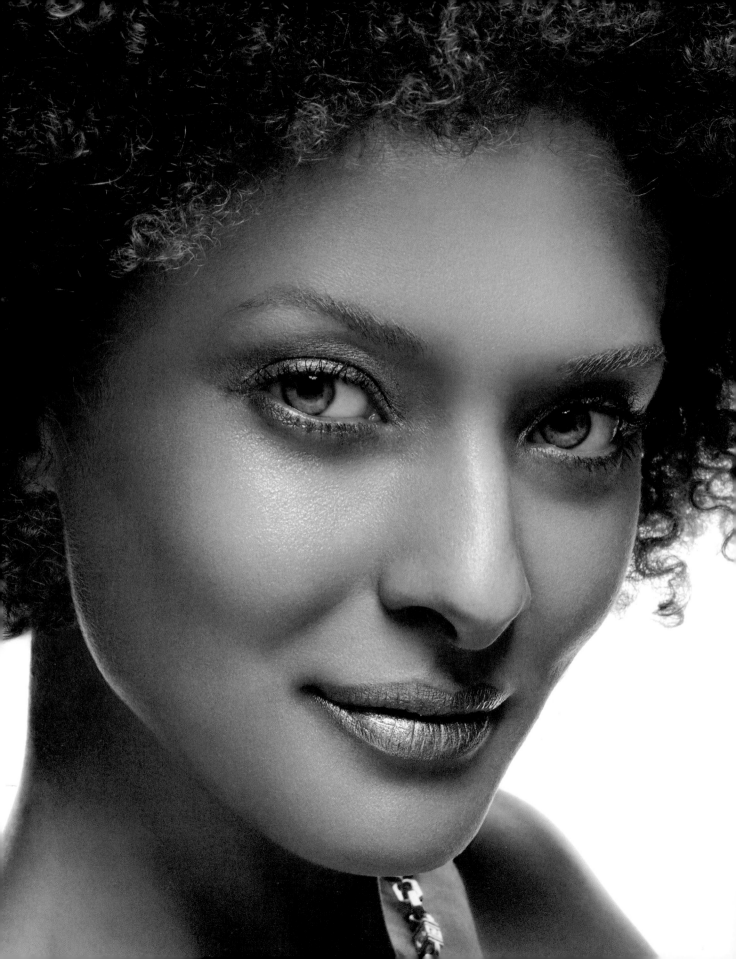

faking it:
high cheekbones

TARTE CHEEK STAIN
IN DOLLFACE

A flush of sheer baby-doll pink adds youth and life to any face. This award-winning push-up stick contains a melt-on-your skin gel formula in a soft, shimmery shade of pink.

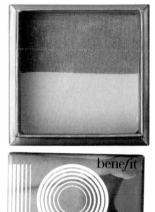

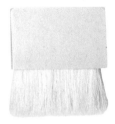

BENEFIT 10

This box of powder scores a perfect ten. One stripe is a golden brown for contouring, the other stripe is a pale pearl pink—with one brush stroke you've highlighted and contoured all at once.

LORAC
LUMINIZER
PEARL L1

Lightly dab this oil-free luminizer onto your temples for an instant cheek pick me-up. The incandescent sheen will draw people's eyes up, making cheekbones appear higher.

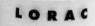

SEPHORA BRAND
PROFESSIONEL PLATINUM
STIPPLING BRUSH

Give cheeks a natural-looking kiss of color with this supersoft brush. The blend of goat hair and high-grade nylon master the art of blending different colors and textures.

FROM ZERO
TO FLAWLESS

Models don't wake up looking like cover girls. Case in point: Our model Tova (pictured) came to our photo shoot in a love-worn sweatshirt, no makeup—albeit with perfect bone structure—and messy hair. Her natural beauty radiated through, but it still took a lot of work to get her in photo-ready shape. On the streets of New York, models go virtually unnoticed. The reason? It takes skilled makeup artists and hair stylists, the right lighting, a genius photographer, and hours of retouching for them to transform into the familiar faces we worship and envy. But be warned: All is not what it seems. "When you look at the airbrushed magazines and advertisements, the models look like aliens when there's not one pore on their face—it's just not normal," says Bare Escentuals CEO Leslie Blodgett. "I would love for pores to make a comeback. There's something sexy about skin that has a little more reveal to it." Imperfections can indeed be charming. Which is why we wanted to show you that imperfect beauty can still be quite beautiful and that "flawless" doesn't always have to be your final destination.

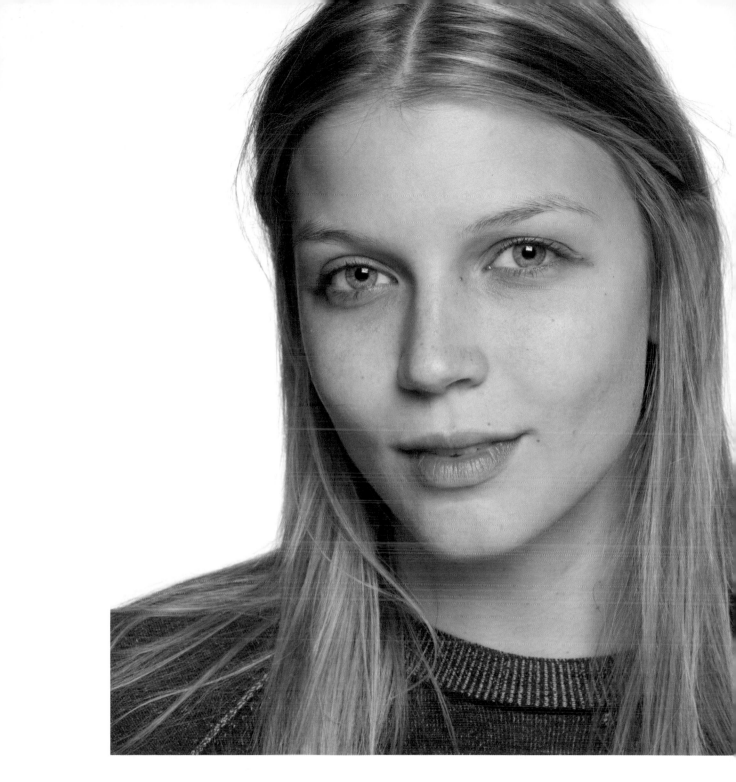

STARTING AT ZERO

Tova, sans a stitch of makeup and with a cup of coffee in hand, entered the photo studio looking like a fresh-faced college student.

HALFWAY THERE

After some concealer, eye shadow, mascara, and a little eyebrow grooming, Tova's looking more glamazon and less undergrad.

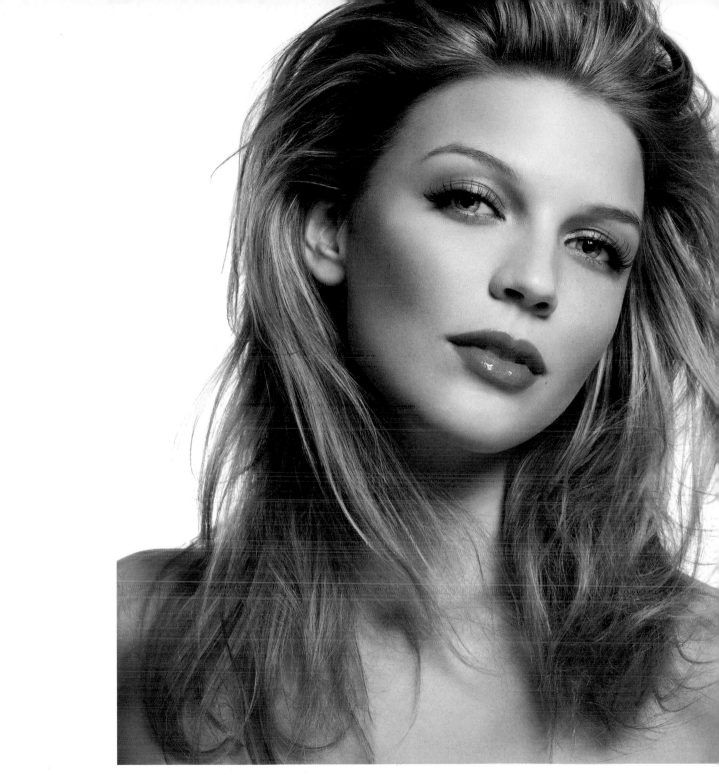

UTTERLY FLAWLESS

Nothing says "cover girl" like glossy, pouty lips, smoky eyes, deeply flushed cheeks, and an übersexy, perfectly tousled coif (wind machine not pictured). It's not easy being flawless . . .

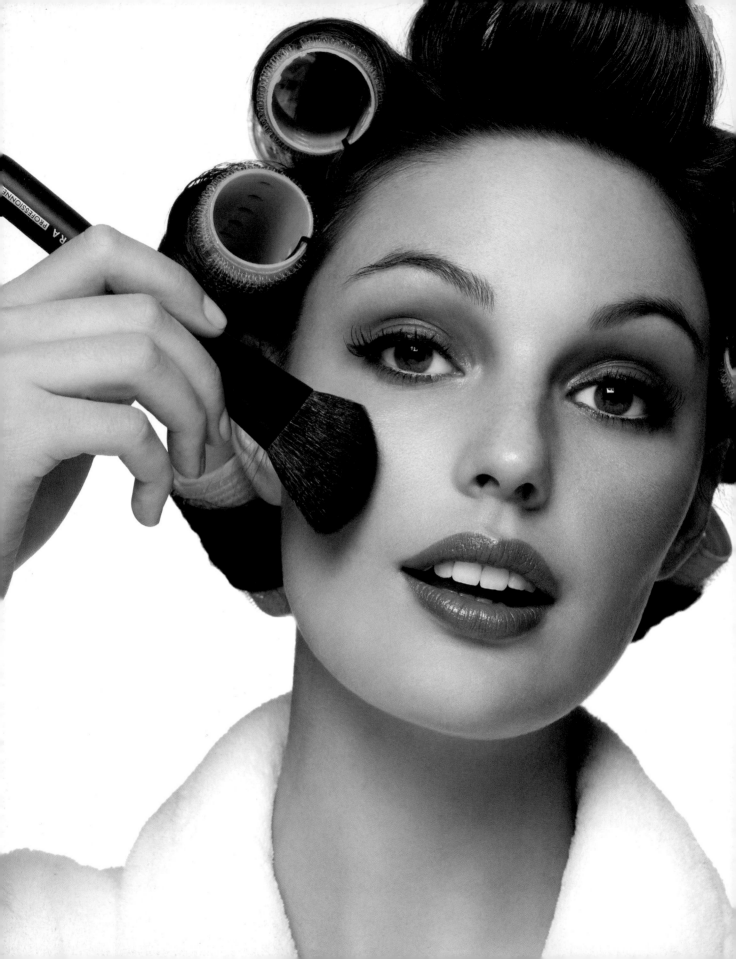

try this at home

We've all seen her. You know the type. Her hair is never out of place—or, if it is, then it's artfully tousled just so. Her brows have that sleek arch to them. Her eye makeup is always sultry, feminine, and chic. She's Ms. Perfect. We kind of hate her, but even more than that, we want to know exactly how she does it. Chances are she had an informed big sister or a very glamorous mother guiding her. We're going to one-up Ms. Perfect, as our beauty experts divulge what it takes to leave the house looking like you have your own team of hair stylists and makeup artists. In this chapter, get all the best tips, tricks, secrets, and advice on what you need to achieve the daunting beauty feats and classic makeup looks you've always wanted to try. Watch your back, Ms. Perfect!

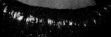

DOUBLEAGENT

DOUBLEAGENT

Use an eye primer on lips to help lipstick stay put.

Dab a gold or pink loose powder onto the center of lips with your finger for a pop of shimmer.

TRY . . . RED LIPS

"Red lips say something very positive about how you feel about yourself," says makeup artist Sue Devitt. Indeed, it takes a bold, confident woman to step out in red lips. Unlike the clear glossophiles, the red-lipsticked among us will get noticed. "Putting on red lipstick instantly transforms your face. It's the quickest way to go from real-life to red-carpet glamour," says LORAC founder Carol Shaw. And one thing's for sure—red lips, like the little black dress, will never go out of style.

get the look

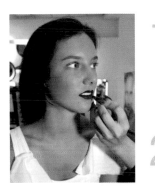

1 Use a lip-toned lip liner to line the true lip line of the mouth. Modifying the lip line when using red lipstick is a big no-no. Feather the lip liner using short strokes and then smudge the line with your fingers to soften it up.

2 Use a lip brush to paint the lip color onto the lips. Smile with the mouth closed and, using a clean eye shadow brush, soften the edges. "I like it when the mouth is diffused, so it looks a little bit out of focus," says Shiseido makeup artist Dick Page.

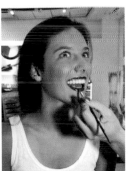

3 Dip the eye shadow brush into flesh-toned pressed powder and follow along the edge of the lip to cover up and remove any imperfections.

words of wisdom

"I love how red lips look on a woman who wears glasses—it creates a beautiful balance."

—Ross Burton

BEAUTY tip

"If you're wearing a turtleneck or a blazer in a deeper color like black, gray, or forest green, red lipstick sets it off beautifully."

—Sue Devitt

"A true red on the lips is so iconic that it registers as a neutral in my mind."

—Dick Page

red between the lines

"Red is sexy and sophisticated—it's extremely feminine and a true classic. The best part is that *anyone* can wear it," says Vincent Longo. "It's just about finding the texture that works for you." Here, the four faces of red:

GLOSS: For just a hint of red and a whole lot of shine, go for gloss. This formula can be used whenever, wherever.

STAIN: The most natural-looking of the bunch. Use your fingers to blend in the stain and you'll get a young, fresh, I-just-ate-a-popsicle look.

SHEER: Great for when you want more than a stain, but aren't ready for full-on fire-engine red. This formula also allows you to build until you reach your desired intensity.

MATTE: The most dramatic red you can get! Save this formula for black tie affairs and evenings when you want your look to be special.

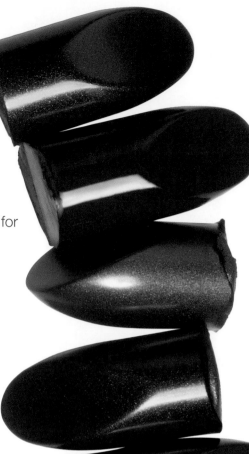
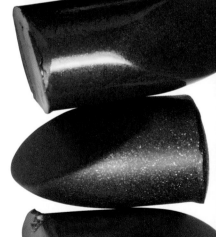
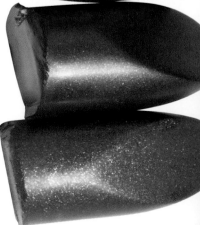

red lip FAQs

Q: I'm all set to wear my red lipstick, but what do I do with the rest of my makeup?

a: Red lips should be the only feature on your face making a statement. Leave everything else light and simple. "It's very chic to pair a red lip with a well-groomed eyebrow, black mascara, and chocolate brown eyeliner," says makeup artist Dick Page. "But to keep it from looking too dragon lady, use a pink blush on the cheeks—it's sophisticated and still has a freshness to it."

Q: What are the biggest mistakes when it comes to wearing red lipstick?

a: "Never apply red lipstick to chapped lips!" says Ross Burton, national artistic director at Lancôme. If your lips are dry, Burton suggests exfoliating them by rubbing gently with a toothbrush and applying a lip balm before the red lipstick. "Another thing that ruins your credibility with red lipstick is bleeding," says DuWop founder Cristina Bartolucci. "Before application, trace all the way around the lips with a neutral lip liner—it acts like a fence for lipstick."

Q: How do I keep my red lipstick from transferring onto everything I kiss, drink, or eat?

a: Blotting is key. After you've applied your lipstick, kiss a tissue or the back of your hand a couple times until no trace of lipstick is left behind. Or if you know you're going to be doing a lot of air-kissing that night, use a red gel-based stain on lips, as opposed to a gloss or lipstick.

BEAUTY secret

Always apply a red stain to the lips before red lipstick. When the color from the lipstick begins to fade, you'll still have a red flush on the lips.

try this at home: red lips

SEPHORA BRAND CREAM LIPSTICK 94

This easy-to-wear classic red hue is the ultimate accessory; it looks gorgeous with jeans as well as a little black cocktail dress. The creamy, rich formula melts onto lips, lasting for hours.

DIOR ROUGE REPLENISHING LIP COLOR IN RED PREMIERE 752

This make-an-entrance hue achieves a lipstick trifecta: stay-on power, complete coverage, and major shine. Layer it on for more intense color.

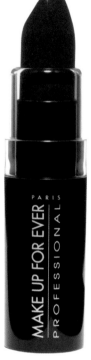

MUFE LIPSTICK IN BLUE RED 205

Blue-reds are universally flattering and this one is a creamy berry that leaves lips silky smooth and dramatic. Bonus: Teeth also look a couple shades whiter against this color.

SEPHORA PROFESSIONEL PLATINUM SQUARE RETRACTABLE LIP BRUSH #60

It's all about a precise application with red lipstick. If your look calls for a drop-dead red, don't leave home without this travel-ready retractable lip brush in your bag.

CARGO REVERSE LIP LINER

This natural-colored pencil adds fullness and definition to lips while locking lip color in place.

TRY . . . EYEBROW SHAPING

Perfectly groomed eyebrows, just like manicured nails, can make a huge difference in presenting yourself as sophisticated, distinguished, and on top of your beauty game. A great pair of eyebrows can even have transformative powers. "People will think you look beautiful without knowing exactly why," says celebrity brow shaper Anastasia Soare. On the flip side, neglected brows can do major damage to your look. "Brows are an essential part of every trend," says Too Faced creator Jerrod Blandino. "When your brows are left ungroomed, it can make your whole appearance look passé." And in beauty, as in fashion, being passé is a serious crime.

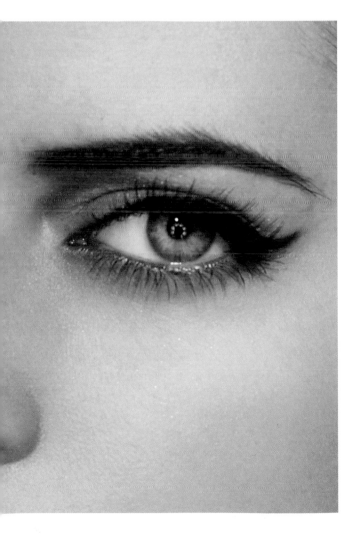

words of wisdom

"As you age, you lose eyebrow hair from the outside in, so the longer your brow is, the younger you look. Use a defining pencil for precision to elongate the brows out toward the temples." —Jerrod Blandino

get the look

Discover your golden arches with these brow-shaping steps:

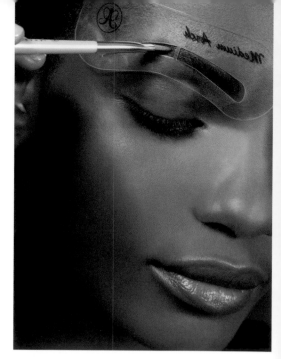

1. First, you'll need a brow stencil. Brow stencils are amazing tools for getting brows to look as if they were shaped by a pro. (Kits from many brands—such as Sephora, Anastasia, Too Faced, and Tarte—include stencils.) To find the stencil that's right for you, Soare suggests taking a pencil and holding it directly up from the center of one of your nostrils. The point where it hits the eyebrow is where the stencil should start. Then hold the pencil diagonally starting at the outside corner of your nose; the point where it hits your brow is where the stencil should end. Repeat with the other nostril.

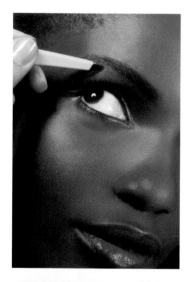

2. Fill in the stencil with a white or pink shadow so it stands out against your natural brow color. Remove the stencil and pluck the area where you don't see eye shadow. "All brows should have somewhat of an arch," says Lancôme's Ross Burton. "When the bone area about two-thirds into and underneath the brow is exposed, it lifts and brightens the entire eye area by allowing light to come in. This effect can shave five years off the appearance."

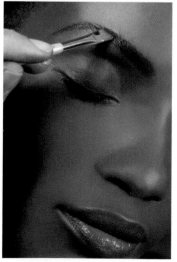

3. Fill in brow hairs with a pencil or powder. Choose a color a shade lighter for darker brows and a shade darker for lighter brows, but be careful not to go too dark, as the oils in your skin collect in your brows and darken the color, making them look artificial.

BROW KNOW-HOW

what's the difference between . . .

BROW WAX Usually clear, brow wax can be used over the natural brow or over pencil or shadow to hold brow hairs in place. Brow wax gives a very natural look. Always use an angled brow brush to apply.

BROW GEL Brow gel can be colored or clear. Brow gel is applied with a spooly brush, just like mascara. Brow gel gives definition to brow hairs by helping them stand up and holding them in place.

BROW PENCIL Brow pencils give precise definition to eyebrows. Pencils are great for achieving subtle, hairlike strokes. Always make sure to sharpen them before use.

BROW POWDER Powder has more pigmentation than pencils, so when you want a more dramatic look, powder is the way to go. Use it wet for maximum intensity. You can mix and match different shades to create the best color for you. An angled brow brush is a must when using powder.

BEAUTY tips

"Eyebrows are sisters, not twins— they do not have to be identical. Everyone has one brow that's higher, so don't become obsessed with making them look exactly alike."

—Ross Burton

"If you're trying to let your brows grow in but still want to groom them, take an old toothbrush and brush the eyebrow hairs all the way up and cut the extra-long hairs sticking up with a tiny pair of professional scissors. You'll get a nice full brow without any tweezing."

—Jane Ford

"Slanted-tip tweezers are much easier to use for plucking brows because the brow bone is curved, and when you're holding the tweezers at a 45-degree angle, they give you great control."

—Anastasia Soare

"Highlighting the arch under the brow with a light eye shadow opens up and lifts the eye immediately."

—Vincent Longo

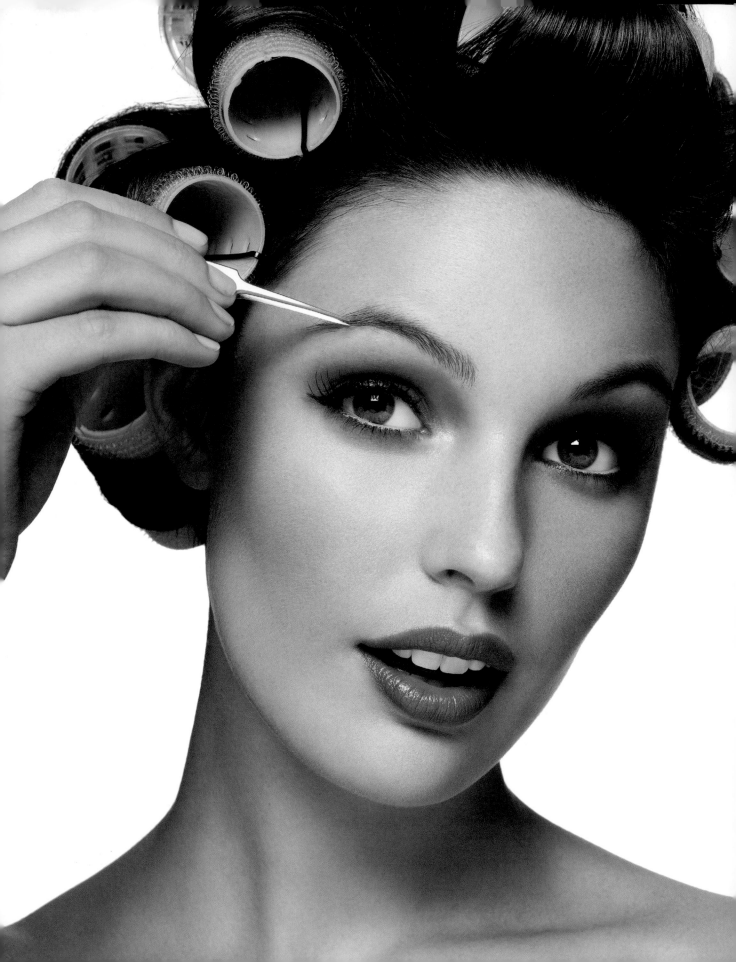

TARTE THE TOOLBOX

This pretty little kit holds all the tools for perfect brows: brow gel, brow pencil, tweezer, brow brush, brow powder, brow wax, and three brow-shaping stencils, plus a compact with a mirror.

TWEEZERMAN PETITE TWEEZER SET

From the top name in tweezers comes this travel-ready set containing two stainless steel tweezers: one slanted tweezer for general tweezing needs, and one superfine, pointed tweezer for more refined tweezing.

BENEFIT SHE-LAQ

No brow hair will ever be out of place thanks to this clear sealant. Use the customized eyebrow brush that's included to brush hairs into perfect place and keep them there.

SEPHORA EYEBROW TRIMMER/BRUSH

Use these eyebrow scissors with a genius comb attachment as a guide to prevent over-trimming. Just comb through brows in the opposite direction of the hair growth and trim the extra-long hairs only.

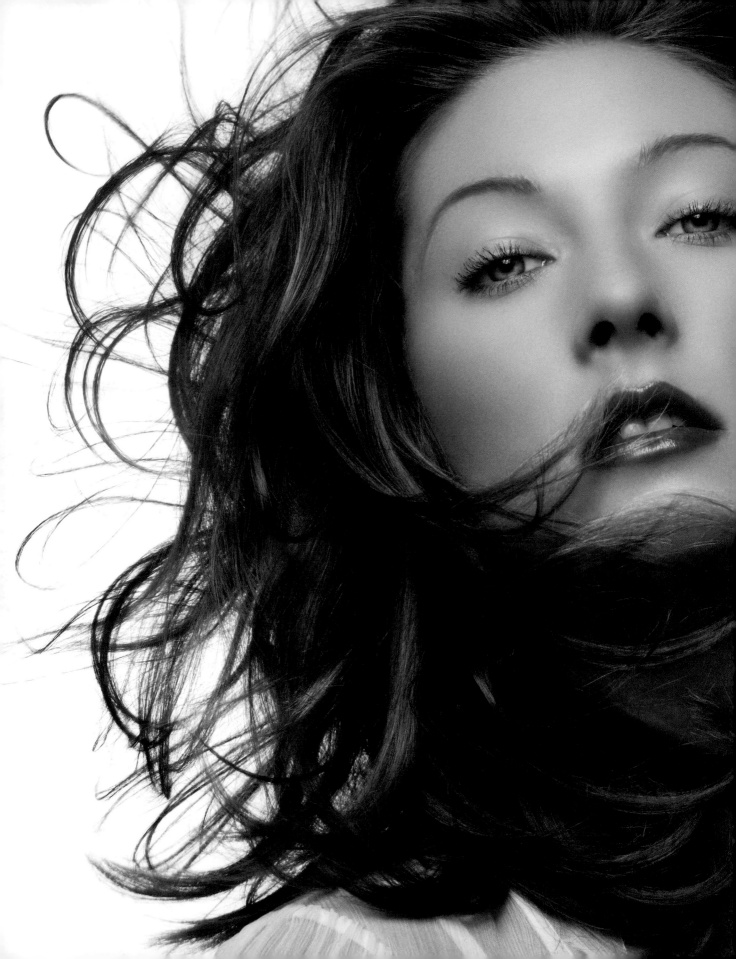

TRY . . . A SALON-STYLE BLOWOUT

It's amazing what a good hair day can do for the psyche. When we look in the mirror and see a cascade of shiny, bouncy hair, suddenly asking for that promotion or striking up a conversation with the cutie in the elevator doesn't seem like such a bad idea. Unfortunately, good hair days, like the weather, are hard to predict. But contrary to what it may seem, a gorgeously styled head of hair isn't derived from a random bout of good luck—it comes from knowing exactly what to do with your wet 'do.

get the look

Follow this formula for salon-perfect hair.

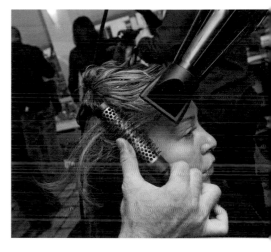

1 Remove excess water from your hair by blotting it with a towel and lightly squeezing, until about 50 percent dry. Apply a quarter-sized amount of straightening product for long hair and a dime-sized amount for short to medium lengths. Comb through with a wide-tooth comb to evenly distribute. "If you put product into soaking-wet hair, the water will dilute it and block it from penetrating into the hair," says Oscar Blandi.

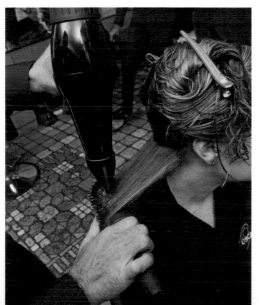

2 Choose a volumizing product for the roots. "Straight doesn't have to mean flat," says Blandi. "No matter what your hair type, everyone looks better with a little body at the roots," agrees Frédéric Fekkai. Spray the volumizer on the crown of the head, covering the area a cap would cover. Using a natural-bristle round brush, lift the face-framing layers of hair up and away from the face, and blow-dry each strand in the opposite direction from which it grows.

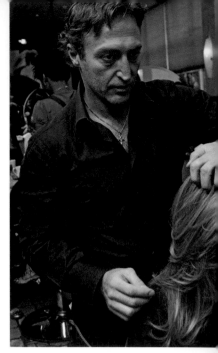

3 Section the rest of the hair into about four different sections, depending on length and thickness, and secure with clips. If you have a lot of hair, there should be three sections on each side of the head: one on top (from the crown to the tops of ears), one in the middle (from ears to jawline) and one for the bottom (jawline to the nape of the neck area).

4 Begin blow-drying the lower sections first. Use a medium- to large-barrel round brush for long hair or small to medium for shorter lengths. Lift the section of hair with the brush and slide it down to the ends, following the strand with the dryer the entire length of the hair. The nozzle attachment that's used to concentrate the air should be pointed down to seal the cuticle, eliminating any frizz. "The hair should never be fully rolled into the brush," says Fekkai. "The brush is only to create tension for the hair." To create that tension, keep the bottom end only of each section rolled into the brush so strands are super-taut. After each strand is dry, do exactly the same movement, but with cold air instead of warm, to close the shaft. For an extra-bouncy, voluminous look, wrap each section in a large Velcro roller after drying, letting it cool in that position for about ten minutes.

5 Finish by rubbing a dollop of silicone serum into your palms and running them down the length of your hair to tame flyaways and add shine.

6 A good blowout should last two to three days. To refresh hair in the mornings without rewashing, mist a brush with water or with a restyling spray, such as Oscar Blandi Jasmine Protein Mist, and restyle the hairline.

BEAUTY tip

"Start fighting frizz in the shower! Don't only rely on a styling aid—choose a shampoo and conditioner regimen designed to eliminate frizz." —Oscar Blandi

words of wisdom

"The best beauty advice I've ever received was to cut my bangs! I finally did it and now I look twenty years younger!" —Anastasia Soare

"I always blow-dry my hair at night, so I'm a lot more relaxed and not in a rush. I sit down in front of a mirror because standing up takes a toll on my arms, and place all the tools on the floor in front of me."
—Gina Bertolotti

"After shampooing, mix two tablespoons of apple cider vinegar and sixteen ounces of mineral water with Fekkai Technician Mask. Pour over the hair, comb it through, and rinse with cold water. The vinegar will close the hair shaft, while the conditioner will smooth and flatten the cuticle." —Frédéric Fekkai

PILLOW TALK

- Silk pillowcases can cause static. Use 500-thread count Egyptian cotton instead.

- Always make sure to change your pillowcase the day after using an overnight hair treatment. The oils and ingredients in the treatment can irritate the skin and cause breakouts.

try this at home:
salon style BLOWOUT

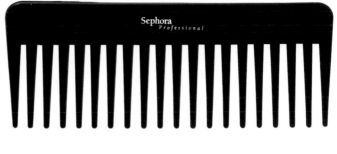

SEPHORA WIDE-TOOTH COMB

Anyone serious about hair care needs to have a wide-tooth comb in her beauty arsenal. Use it to comb conditioner and treatment products evenly from roots to ends, or to divide hair into sections for a perfect blow-dry.

OSCAR BLANDI LUCE

This rinse-out gloss infuses shine into even the dullest of hair. Leave it on for 3 to 5 minutes after shampooing and conditioning.

FEKKAI COIF IRONLESS STRAIGHTENING BALM

Professional relaxing treatments can be expensive, time-consuming, and terrible for the hair. Instead, go for this chemical-free straightening balm, which is nothing short of miraculous. It gets locks pencil-straight and leaves them silky smooth and strengthened.

OSCAR BLANDI NO GRAVITY

Everyone looks better with volume at the roots. Blandi says to apply this product onto roots before blow-drying hair, then flip your head upside-down and use your fingers to open up sections while applying heat.

TRY . . . SMOKY EYES

"When you see a woman with a smoky eye who normally doesn't wear much eye makeup, there's always a wow factor," says DuWop cofounder Cristina Bartolucci. Nothing's sultrier or sets the eyes off better than a smudgy, smoldering, smoky eye. This is the one makeup trick every woman should master for maximum sex appeal.

get the look

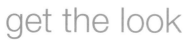

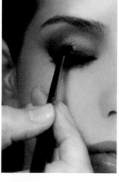

1 Apply an eye shadow primer onto lids and below the lower lashline to prevent color from creasing or running. Sweep a shade a little lighter than flesh tone onto entire lid, from brow to lashline.

2 Choose the color you want to smoke out with. "Take any color you want and blend it with some black eye shadow for an instantly smoky shade," says LORAC founder and celebrity makeup artist Carol Shaw. Apply your chosen color from the lashline up to the crease and smudge in a little black eye shadow over it with your finger. Use a larger eye shadow brush to blend both colors together.

3 Line the outer third of the upper lashline with a black pencil, then go over that line with a smudge brush dipped in the eye shadow you just used to smoke out the eye.

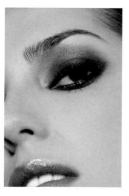

4 Line the lower lashline. "Rather than using horizontal strokes to apply the liner on the lower lashline, try using a very small brush with tiny vertical strokes," says Vincent Longo. Dip the brush in the color, then hold the brush vertical against your lashline and with vertical strokes, move along your lashline. "It will give you a baby-soft smoky blend and it keeps the intensity of the color very close to the root of the lash, so you get the smoky effect without looking too overdone," explains Longo. For a variation on the classic, Longo loves plum mixed with brown. He suggests using a brown pencil first followed by an application of plum eye shadow over the pencil.

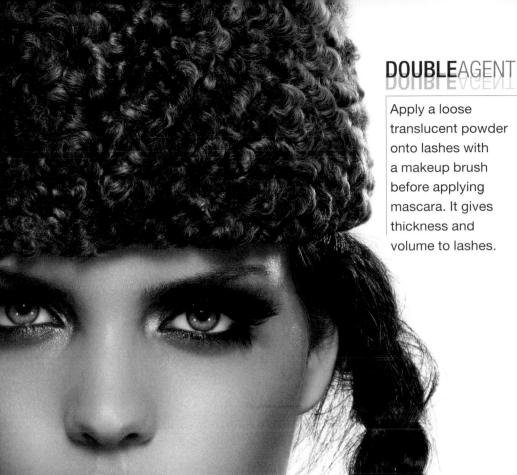

DOUBLEAGENT

Apply a loose translucent powder onto lashes with a makeup brush before applying mascara. It gives thickness and volume to lashes.

5 "What grounds a smoky eye is lashes," says Bartolucci. "Otherwise it can look like a black eye." She suggests curling lashes, then applying anywhere from two to six coats of mascara, combing out the lashes in between each coat.

BEAUTY SCHOOL: EYELINER
master the technique of a perfect line

"Aim to apply your eyeliner at the root of the eyelash," says Laura Geller. "The goal is to get the line so close to the lashline that it looks more like a backing to your lash. When you see even a little bit of skin between the line and your lashline, it's obvious." For an almost invisible line, Gellar suggests sharpening your pencil until the point is super-thin and resting the point on the base of the lash so you're actually touching where the lash grows. With very gentle, short strokes, create a line on your upper lashes.

hues for you

Dior global makeup advisor Shane Paish chooses his favorite smoky eye shades:

BLUE EYES: Slate grays and purple-based browns
BROWN EYES: Chestnuts, burgundies, warm beiges, and taupes
GREEN EYES: Colors with a warm orange base tone

BEAUTY tips

"Apply your makeup standing up! When you're standing, as opposed to sitting at a makeup mirror hunched over a cup of coffee, you'll be more serious and you'll apply like a pro."

—Jean Ford

"I have brown eyes and whenever I wear green shadow, people stop and ask me if I've been on vacation. It makes the eyes pop and gives an all-over glow to the complexion."

—Hana Zalzal

STILA SMUDGE POTS

This inky gel holds the key to smoldering eyes. Smudge it with your finger close to the lash line for a smoky intensity.

BENEFIT BAD GAL LASH

The ultimate smoky eye companion. This chunky wand of mascara delivers full, sexy lashes in a single stroke.

LORAC STARRY EYED BAKED EYE SHADOW TRIO IN RISING STAR

LORAC founder and makeup artist to the stars Carol Shaw designed this shimmering trio of perfectly matched metallic shadows herself. The shades were baked on a terracotta disk to ensure a glamorous, long-wearing smoky eye.

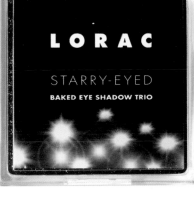

URBAN DECAY PRIMER POTION

This magic wand is eyeshadow's best friend. You can cry, swim, or shower and any shadow you've applied over this invisible potion won't crease or budge.

STILA SMOKY EYE TALKING PALETTE

Just like having your own makeup instructor, this palette of four smoky shades talks you through the steps you need to achieve a perfect smoky eye. Just press the button and a Stila artist's voice comes on with directions.

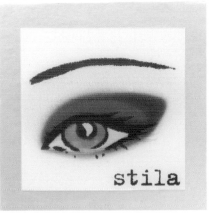

BEAUTY
tip

"Blue mascara really flatters the eyes—it makes the whites look brighter and it's a really fun way to wear color with low commitment."

—Wende Zomnir

SEPHORA

TRY . . . FAKE LASHES

Take a deep breath and say: "I can apply fake lashes." You *can* and you *should.* Forget any preconceived notion about fake lashes looking, well, fake. When done correctly, they can add major volume to your lashes, open up the eyes, and transform you into a serious glamazon. What's more, they make all your other makeup look better. Fake lashes and mascara are like peanut butter and jelly—alone they're just fine, but when you put the two together, unbelievable magic happens.

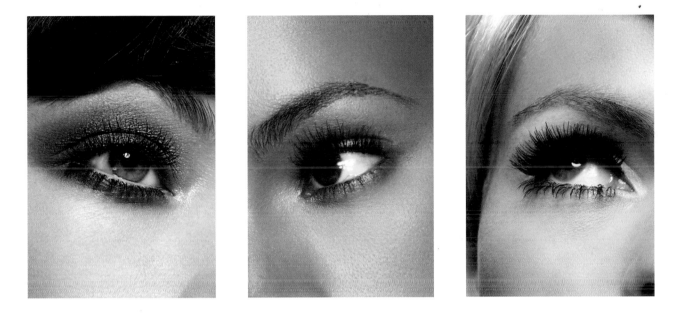

BEAUTY tip

"When wearing fake lashes, always carry a little bit of adhesive and a toothpick with you. If the lash starts to come loose, hold the toothpick with the adhesive on it onto the root of the lash until it feels secure."

—Laura Geller

get the look

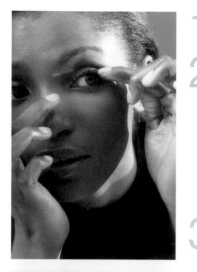

1 Curl your lashes.

2 Apply an oblong bead of adhesive glue onto the length of the lash strip. Strips come in various different sizes, from a full set of lashes to singlets. If you're working with a full strip, cut it in half. It's much less difficult to work with a half strip, while single lashes are the easiest to maneuver. Use a gel-based glue as opposed to latex, which can create a film on the lid.

3 Let the glue dry for a few seconds before you apply the lashes so it becomes tacky; this makes application easier. Tilt your head back a bit and apply the lashes with tweezers, aiming for the center of your upper lashline. Get right into the lashline so there is no space between the falsies and your natural lashes. "Try to keep looking down until the glue has set to avoid getting glue onto your eyelids," advises Bourjois makeup artist Melissa Silver. Make any adjustments before the glue sets.

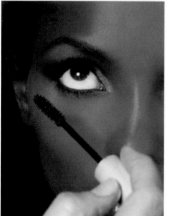

4 Go over your lashline with a thin line of liquid liner if you see any spaces between your lashline and the false lashes.

5 Curl the combination of your natural lashes with the false lashes.

6 Apply mascara, grabbing the false lashes and your natural lashes through the wand together. "The mascara will gel them together, giving you a unified look," says Vincent Longo.

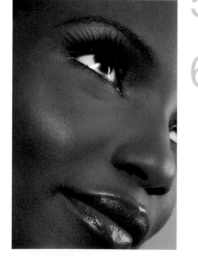

try this at home:
fake LASHES

FIBERWIG BLACK MASCARA

There's much buzz surrounding this new mascara from Japan. And with good reason! The formula is engineered to create ideal lashes by imparting a perfect, smudge-proof maximum lash extension effect with a water-resistant formula that's easy to remove with warm water, without risking, damaging, or losing your natural lashes.

SEPHORA EYE LASH CURLER

Pinch-proof and foolproof, this classic lash curler is a must for every makeup kit. Stash one at home, the office, and in your purse for a wide-eyed, beautiful look 24/7.

SEPHORA LASH PLACEMENT KIT

Take the one-handed approach to false lash application with this easy-to-use lash-placing tool. The contoured tip provides the perfect placement of lashes and removes them with ease. To use: Gently grasp false lashes at the lashline with the tip; apply a thin line of lash adhesive to the lash band. Let dry a few seconds until tacky, close eyelid, then press the soft-tipped applicator just above natural lashes.

MAKE UP FOR EVER FALSE EYELASHES

Add a hint of cat-eyed flirtiness to your wink with these professional-quality lashes. Use them to give just a little lift to the outer corners of eyes, or all around the eye for full-on drama.

LORAC FRONT OF THE LINE WATERPROOF EYELINER

Steady hand no longer required in order to achieve a clean, precise line. The flexible tip on this waterproof eyeliner provides smooth strokes and ultimate control, so you can go from very fine to dramatically bold in one stroke.

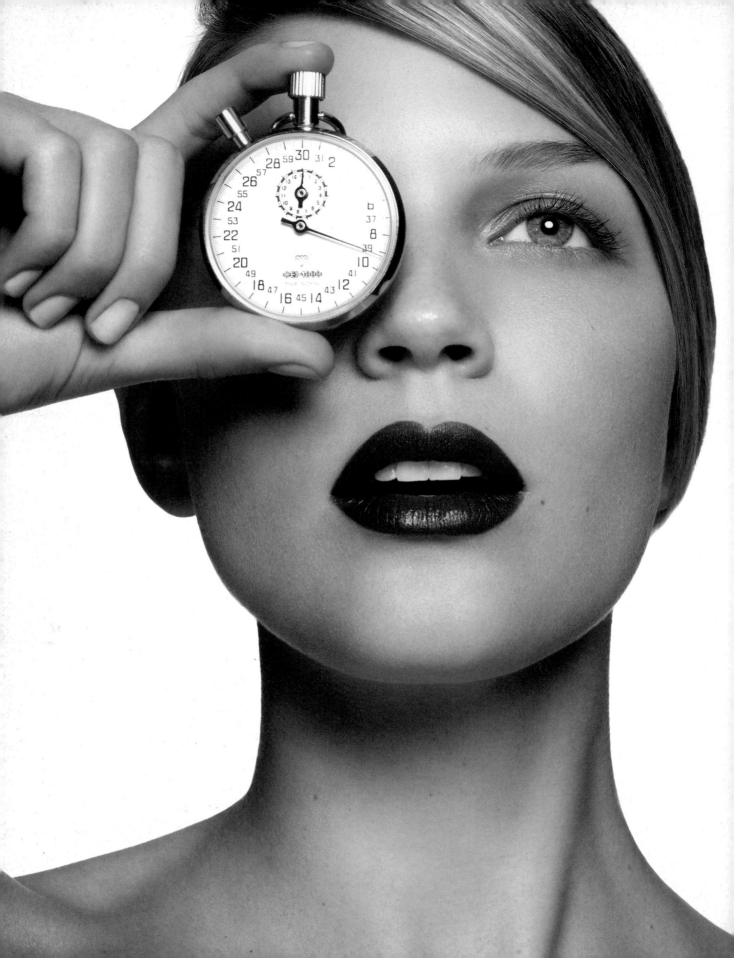

quick fixes

Oops, you did it again. That dollop of pomade was way too generous. Will you ever learn? Now you have a few options. Option one: Tell people you're trying to revive the grunge look and leave your hair stringy and matted to your scalp. Option two: Re-shower and be an hour late to your meeting. Option three: Fix it with one of the tricks you'll learn in this chapter. If you've ever ruined what was becoming a flawless makeup application by putting way too much concealer on a zit or by creating lashes so clumpy they could be used as pipe cleaners, you've come to the right place. First we'll teach you how to fix it, then we'll teach you how to prevent it from happening next time. Buh-bye, beauty boo-boos!

FIX . . . CAKED-ON CONCEALER

You made a mountain out of that molehill of a zit on your cheek. Now what? "Too much concealer on a blemish is going to give the illusion of volume," says Ross Burton, makeup artist and national artistic director at Lancôme. "Take a tissue and slightly buff the concealer away. If the pimple still has too much product on it, moisten a cotton swab with makeup remover and dab at it until it no longer rivals Mt. Vesuvius in height. Now you need to re-cover it. Find a concealer brush with a pointy, ultra-fine tip, and lightly touch a bit of concealer onto the redness of the zit—not onto any of the raised area—until you've hidden any discoloration. Then set with a dab of translucent powder.

avoid the mistake

News flash! Concealer is always to be applied *after* foundation. Otherwise it will only get wiped off. And don't expect it to perform miracles. It's called concealer—not disappearer. "Think of concealer as getting rid of the discoloration of the blemish, not of the blemish itself," says makeup artist Laura Geller. In other words, the best it can do is smooth out the color—applying more and more product to it will only call attention to the new frenemy on your face. Another no-no is choosing the wrong color cover-up. "Don't use a concealer color that's too light; otherwise, you'll be highlighting the pimple," says Dick Page, makeup artist and artistic director for Shiseido The Makeup.

Pimples are also much more noticeable when they're shiny and have a reflection to them, so the finish should always be matte. "Matte it with blotting papers or a loose powder to prevent any oil from coming through, which can also dissolve the concealer," says Page. But that said, if the zit in question is dry and cracked, dab it with a little oil-free moisturizer before covering it. After applying the concealer with a fine-tipped concealer brush, blend it with your finger by using a tapping, not wiping, motion. Finally, layer translucent powder over the area with a puff, very gently so as not to pull off any of the carefully laid product you just applied.

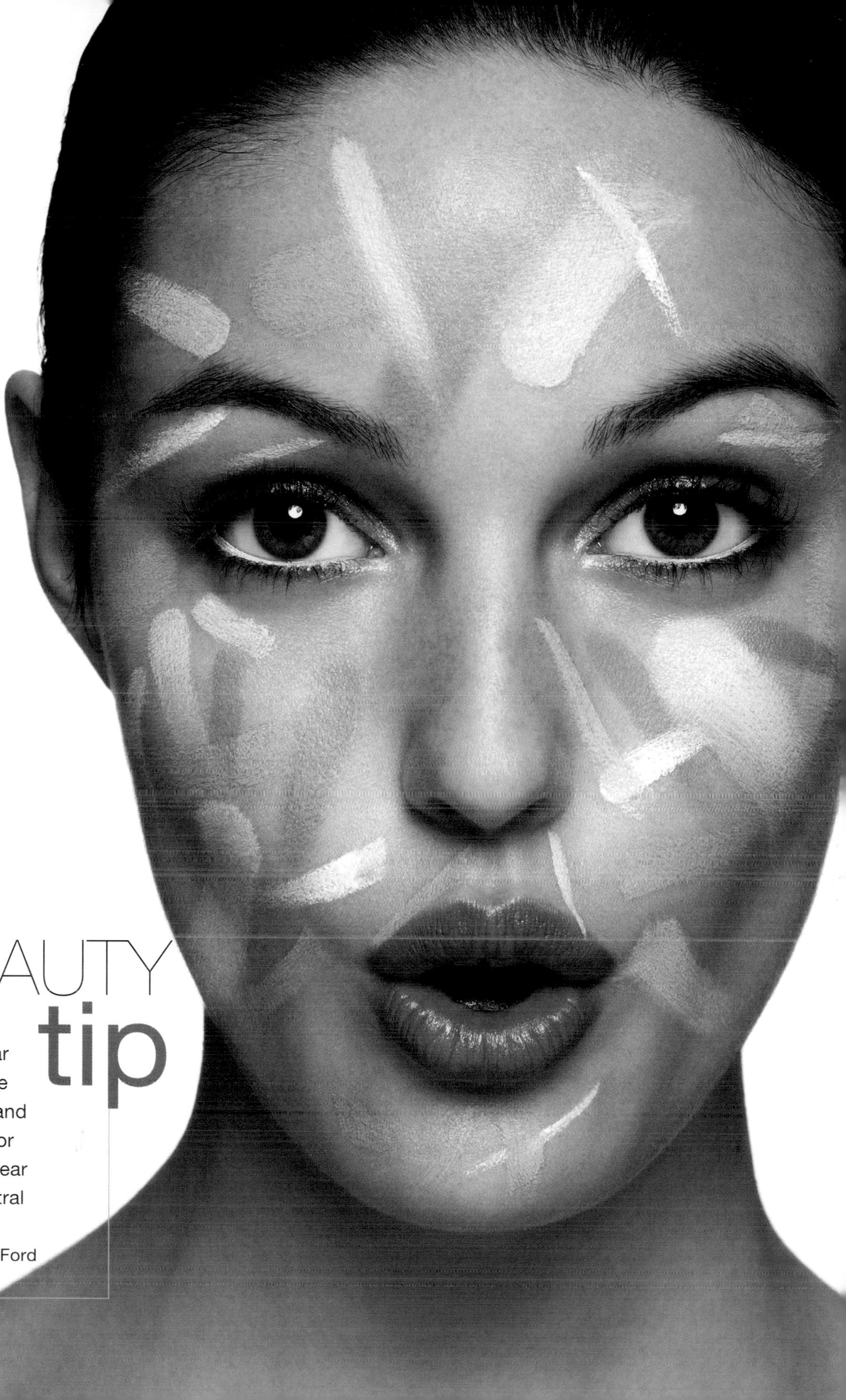

BEAUTY
tip

"If you have a bad
breakout, don't wear
red lipstick, because
you'll be repeating and
bringing out the color
of the blemishes. Wear
a soft brown or neutral
color instead."

—Jane Ford

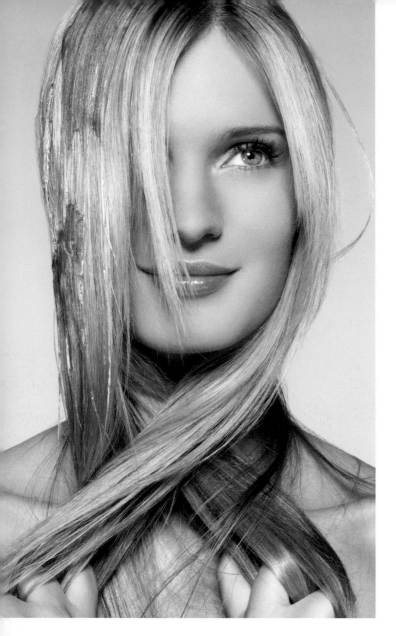

FIX . . . HAIR PRODUCT OVERDOSE

If the product you just OD'd on is oil-based (i.e., serum, styling cream, pomade, shine spray) and you over-applied onto dry hair, douse the spot with baby powder or a dry shampoo. If you've used too much hairspray or gel, the best thing to do is to zap it with blow-dryer heat. If you start to see smoke, don't be alarmed. You're not scorching your locks; it's just the product burning off.

avoid the mistake

"The biggest error I see people make is putting product on the top of the head," says Frédéric Fekkai. "Always apply it to the back first, that's where the density of the hair is, and use what's left over on your hands for the rest of the head." Fekkai suggests using a quarter-sized amount for long hair and pea-sized for short to medium lengths.

FIX . . . FOUNDATION FACE

At best, foundation is an invisible layer that hides any imperfections, smoothes out discoloration, and creates a seamless look on your face. At worst, it can look like a thick mask of makeup. You know you've made a foundation faux pas if your complexion doesn't come close to resembling the texture of your natural skin or if you can see the dreaded line of demarcation anywhere on your face, especially on your jaw. If it's the former, here's what to do: "After the application, wet your fingertips a tiny bit and run them over your face so you don't see any real texture," says makeup artist Victoria Jackson.

Another way to tone down foundation overload is to apply a dime-sized amount of moisturizer onto a foundation brush and work the brush over your face. "It should make the foundation less visible and more complexion-like," says Burton. Another trick up Burton's sleeve for foundation-happy types? "Separate a two-ply tissue in half. Place one ply right on top of the face and move it around really gently with your hand. This will remove any extra foundation."

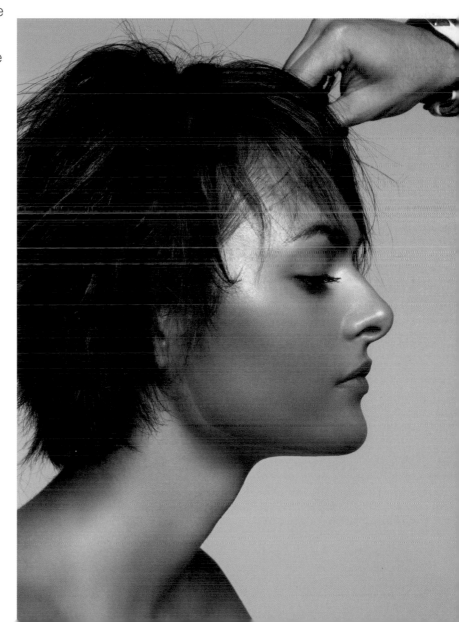

avoid the mistake

1 Always start with a primer! "Primer smoothes out any texture or dry areas on the face," says makeup artist Vincent Longo. "It allows for a very smooth foundation application and the blend becomes much easier." Primer is also like Krazy Glue for foundation; it prevents it from seeping into pores and from melting off in heated situations.

2 Get ready to apply. Start with a quarter-sized amount of foundation; you can always add more. You don't have to do a full face either—just concentrate on blotchy areas and spots that need concealing. "I like to put liquid foundation in the palm of my hand first because the warmth of my skin makes the product more blendable," says Burton.

3 Apply! Work in an area that has exposure to sun and daylight. "Ideally, do it with a window behind you, a mirror in front of you, and the light coming in over your shoulder," says Page. Start in the center of your face and blend in a downward motion toward the jawline, with small, flicking strokes. Always try to follow the grain of the facial hair so the hairs will lay flat against the skin. The entire time you're applying, continue to blend after each stroke. "Many women have a 'makeup face' when they look in the mirror, but that's not how you are in the world, where your face is mobile and active," says Page. He suggests smiling and opening your mouth really wide while you're blending.

how to choose your foundation match

- Liquid/Cream Foundations: Find three foundations you think might be perfect matches. Use a Q-tip to make three different swipes onto your jawline (the area on your face that's least likely to have been touched by sun or environmental damage). Find an area that has direct daylight exposure and look in the mirror. The one that disappears into the skin is your winner.

- Powder Foundations: Rub it into your forearm. The color should disappear into the skin.

decoding foundation formulas

LIQUID

Coverage: Light to medium
Best suited for: All skin types
What it does: Evens out skin tone, leaves a dewy or matte finish depending on the formulation
How to apply it: Use a makeup sponge or foundation brush for fuller coverage, your fingers for lighter coverage

MINERAL

Coverage: Medium
Best suited for: All skin types, but especially good for sensitive, acne-prone, and those with rosacea
What it does: Absorbs oil, moisturizes dry spots, protects skin, and creates an airbrushed look with minerals that have been finely ground into a creamy loose powder
How to apply it: Buff it on with a kabuki brush

STICK

Coverage: Medium to heavy
Best suited for: Combination and oily skin

What it does: Conceals discoloration and imperfections, evens out skin tone
How to apply it: Dab on where you need the most coverage and blend out from there, using fingers or a sponge
Added bonus: Great for travel and on-the-go touch-ups

CREAM TO POWDER

Coverage: Medium
Best suited for: Combination and oily skin types
What it does: Absorbs oil, imparts a natural look with a soft matte finish
How to apply it: Use fingers or a sponge and apply to entire face

TINTED MOISTURIZER

Coverage: Sheer to light
Best suited for: Normal skin types
What it does: Leaves a natural, no-makeup look
How to apply it: Use fingers to blend evenly all over the face

POWDER

Coverage: Light to medium
Best suited for: Oily skin types
What it does: Absorbs oil leaving a matte finish, evens out skin tone, conceals imperfections
How to apply it: Use a dome-shaped brush and sweep onto face in a circular motion

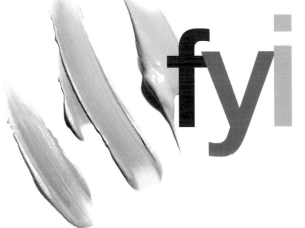

fyi

THE LOWDOWN ON COLOR-CORRECTING PRIMERS

Green = neutralizes redness, rosacea, blemishes
Orange/Peach = neutralizes blue, blue under-eye circles, blue bruises; can also be used to brighten sallow skin
Purple/Lavender = neutralizes yellow, sallowness
Yellow = neutralizes purple under-eye circles, purple bruises; also used to correct mild redness

FIX . . . MASCARA MISHAP

If you've put too much mascara on your lashes, douse a toothbrush with eye-makeup remover and then gently go over the lashes with it. Use a Q-tip that's been hit with remover and then lightly dab any area on the lid that was marred by runaway mascara.

avoid the mistake

1 Just like your skin needs primer pre-foundation, the lashes really benefit from a mascara primer. "Many things happen when you use a lash primer," says makeup artist Laura Geller. "Because most primers are very moisturizing, your mascara will go on less clumpy. Primers can also make lashes look more voluminous, so you'll need a lot less mascara in general. Plus, lashes tend to curl a lot better when you've used a primer."

2 Curl lashes. "Never curl lashes when there's mascara on them," says Geller. "The lashes are drier and very breakable when they have mascara on them, and you are bending the lash in a way that's unnatural."

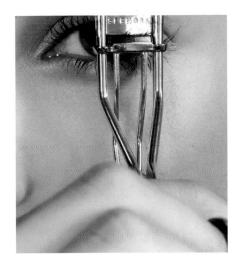

3 Apply mascara. Set the mascara wand at the base of your lashes and wiggle it back and forth through the lashes. "You want the premier deposit to be on the lashline and not the tips," says Benefit cofounder Jane Ford.

4 "You always want to look straight ahead when applying mascara; otherwise, it may end up on your lid," says makeup artist Sue Devitt. "Focus on something straight ahead while lashes are midway open." Another foolproof way to avoid getting any mascara on your eyelid is by relying on a standby office supply. "Take one of those mini Post-it notes and lay it down over your eyelid before applying mascara," says DuWop founder and celebrity makeup artist Cristina Bartolucci.

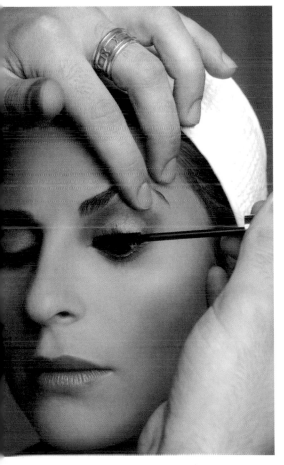

5 Immediately comb out lashes with a spooly brush or lash comb following the application. The key is to get in there with the comb before the mascara has a chance to dry.

fyi

"The reason women always open their mouths when applying mascara is because when your jaw drops, your eyes open."
—Jean Ford

DOUBLE AGENT QUICK FIXES

- Toilet paper instead of blotting paper

- A knife instead of a mirror to check your lipstick

- Nail polish to prevent a run from spreading in your stockings

- Toothbrush as an eyebrow groomer

- Hair conditioner as shaving cream

- Matchbook cover as a nail file

- Brow tint to cover gray hairs or as a root touch-up in between a visit to the colorist

- Pressed or loose powder on roots of hair to absorb grease

- Hand lotion to fight the frizzies

- Cold tea bags to depuff eyes

- Olive oil on patches of ultradry skin

words of wisdom

"The best quick fix in the world is a new tube of lipstick. Unlike fashion, you don't have to worry about it fitting you. A new color of lipstick will instantaneously change your look and lift your spirits."

—Laura Geller

quick FIXES

OSCAR BLANDI PRONTO

Pronto means quick, and that's exactly how this verbena-scented translucent hair powder works. It will extend your blowout, absorb oil on the roots, and help with any product overdose.

LORAC OIL-FREE NEUTRALIZER

This miracle makeup corrects and conceals uneven skin tone in a flash. Infused with natural botanicals, it calms irritated skin, neutralizes redness, and conceals blemishes.

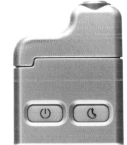

DUWOP SUB-SURFACE

This double-duty product includes a hydrating under-eye primer and a blemish treatment.

ZENO PRO ACNE CLEARING DEVICE

Use this hand-held, FDA-cleared blemish zapper at the first sign of a pimple to fade or disappear your spot within just twenty-four hours. Apply the metal pad directly onto the pimple, leaving it there for 2½ minutes.

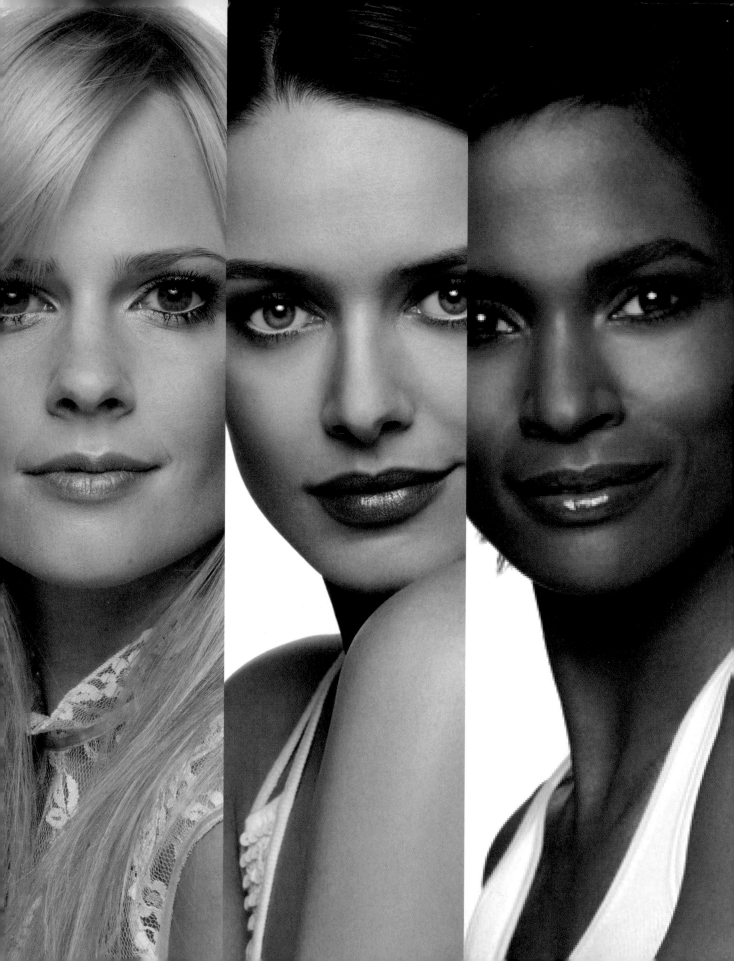

skin
smarts

The secret to obtaining gorgeous, glowing, youthful skin for as long as possible comes with using the right products and by being aware of four major elements: sleep, smoking, the sun, and stress. Sleep is your friend, while the other three are terrorists on your health and complexion. "If you really want to age yourself, go into the sun, smoke a cigarette, and stay up all night," says Dr. Fredric Brandt. But if you're looking to do the opposite, adopt a daily skin care regimen tailor-made for your skin type and practice the safe skin tips in this chapter.

BEAUTY
tip

"Wear pinks! Sheer
pink eye shadows,
soft pink blushes
and pink lipsticks
instantaneously make
you look brighter,
more radiant, and
extraordinarily
youthful."

—Laura Geller

COMPLEXION PERFECTION

do you know your skin type? identify it here:

You have Normal Skin if you have . . .

- An even complexion
- Pores that are normal size
- Skin with very few lines and wrinkles

Your goal is to: Maintain and protect

You have Oily Skin if you have . . .

- An all-over shine
- Pores that are open
- Blackheads, whiteheads, and blemishes
- A sallow appearance
- Few lines and wrinkles

Your goal is to: Minimize shine and make the pores less visible

You have Combination Skin if you have . . .

- An oily T-zone
- Optimal to dry skin on cheeks
- Breakouts on the chin
- Enlarged pores on the chin

Your goal is to: Control oil, normalize the skin, and protect

You have Dry Skin if you have . . .

- Fine, almost invisible pores
- Skin that looks and feels dry, tight, or parched
- A ruddy appearance
- Cheeks that are flaky and dry
- Visible lines and wrinkles around the eyes and mouth

Your goal is to: Hydrate, treat, nourish, and protect

BEAUTY secret

"Whenever I break out, I put some Visine on a spoon, pop it in the freezer for a bit, and then place it on the pimple. It eliminates redness and reduces swelling like magic!"

—Maureen Kelly

every good skin care regimen should look like this:

step 1: Cleanse

Find a cleanser that works with your skin type and wash your face twice a day, in the morning and evening.

step 2: Exfoliate

Slough off dead skin cells at least once a week to pave the way for better absorption.

step 3: Treat

Whether you're concerned with acne, wrinkles, dullness, hyperpigmentation, or all of the above, treat your skin with products that contain specific ingredients to solve every problem.

step 4: Hydrate

Soothe and soften skin immediately after showering for maximum hydration.

step 5: Protect with Sun Care

No matter what your skin type or concerns, protect your skin from future sun and environmental damage with an antioxidant-packed moisturizer and a serious SPF.

skin-care tips for each decade

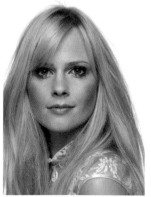

YOUR 20s

- "Eye cream is key in your twenties," says Ole Henriksen. "Purchase one that's rich in texture and extend it out to the temple area, where fine lines are the first to form."
- Cell turnover begins to slow and dead skin cells are not as easily shed, which can lead to a dull, lifeless complexion. Exfoliating products will help slough off the dead cells and reveal the fresh, healthy skin underneath.
- "Eat foods rich in antioxidants, essential fatty acids, and amino acids to increase the hydration of your skin," says Dr. Murad.

YOUR 30s

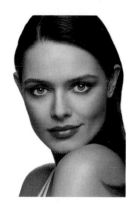

- "Your skin is just beginning to show signs of wrinkles and irregular pigmentation at this age," says Dr. Murad. "It's important to use products with antioxidants topically and internally to help minimize future damage."
- "Invest in a serum and use it prior to your night cream," says Ole Henriksen.
- "Start using products with milder anti-inflammatories like DMAE and phytonutrients such as green tea and olive oil," says Dr. Perricone.

YOUR 40s, 50s, AND BEYOND

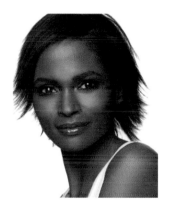

- "In your forties and fifties, you're hitting perimenopause and menopause, where hormonal changes in the body begin to show up on the skin. The skin starts to thin, become dull and dry, and fine lines appear, while excess facial hair and breakouts occur. I call this hormonal aging," says Dr. Murad. "Look for ingredients such as soy, wild yam, clover, and chaparral extract. Use peptides to encourage the minimizing of the fine lines and wrinkles."
- "This is the time to get more aggressive with the more powerful antioxidants, such as alpha lipoic acid, vitamin C ester, and tocotrienols, and neuropeptides," says Dr. Perricone.

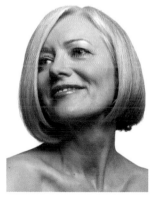

DOUBLE AGENT

Eye cream can also be used on the skin around the lips to prevent fine lines.

skin FAQs

Q: Do I really need to invest in an eye cream? Or can I just use my regular face cream around the eyes?

a: Eye cream is a vital part of every skin care regimen for many reasons. The eye area is the first spot on the face to show aging. Normal skin is around two millimeters thick, but eyelid skin is only 0.5 millimeters thick. So eye creams, which tend to be more emollient than most face creams, will work to keep that area extra-moisturized. Also, your regular face cream may have ingredients in it that will irritate the sensitive eye area. The best way to apply eye cream is with the ring finger, to ensure that you use a light touch. "You only need to apply eye cream around the orbital bone and not any closer to the actual eye, because over time the cream will migrate," explains Dr. Murad. For ultimate protection, invest in an eye cream with SPF.

Q: Why is cleansing my face in the morning important? I made sure it was squeaky clean before I went to sleep . . .

a: "Cleansing in the morning removes any sebum built up during the night and provides an absorbable base for the active ingredients you'll be applying in the morning, including sunscreens," says Dr. Sobel.

Q: What are the major causes of acne?

a: "The causes of acne are multifactorial," says Dr. Perricone. "Hormonal changes in teens can precipitate acne, as can poor diet and stress. A pro-inflammatory diet causes inflammation, which results in clogged pores." Dr. Perricone suggests a diet rich in fresh fruit, vegetables, and coldwater fish. All contain antioxidants to promote healthy skin and bodies. "Stress is also a huge cause of acne," adds Dr. Perricone. "One way it does this is by elevating levels of cortisol, a stress hormone, and other adrenal steroids can act as androgens and stimulate the sebaceous glands, resulting in a flare-up of acne."

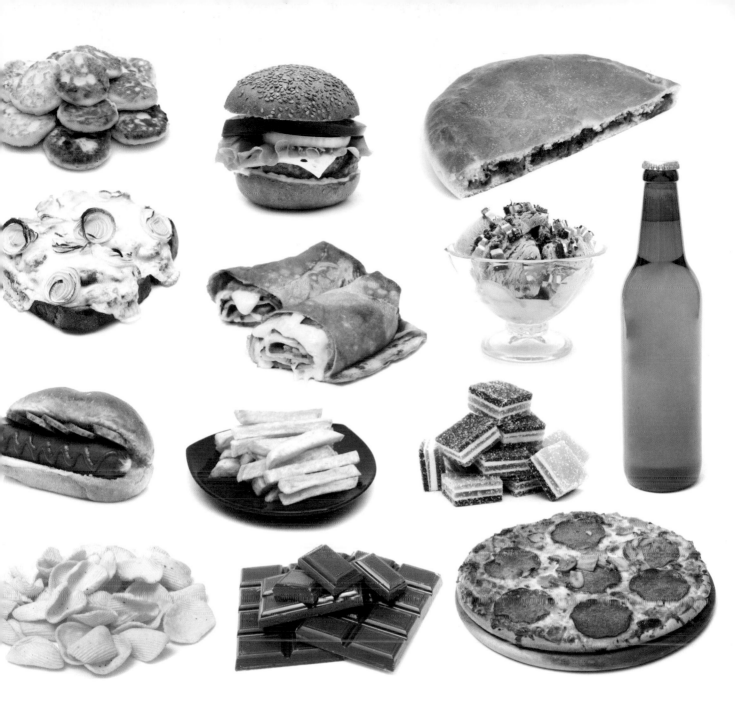

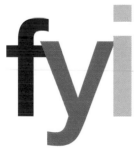 Processed food isn't just fattening—it's also bad for your skin. "Any food that's high in saturated or trans fats and sugars will have a tremendously negative effect on the skin, because it is pro-inflammatory and will cause changes within the pore, resulting in acne," says Dr. Perricone.

words
of wisdom

"Cleaning your face before you go to sleep is so important because not only are you removing makeup, but you're also washing off any harmful pollutants that may have landed on your skin throughout the day."

—Dr. Howard Murad

SLEEPING BEAUTY

Anyone who has ever taken the red-eye knows how important a good night's sleep is to feeling beautiful. "Cellular repair takes place while we sleep, resulting in smoother, more radiant skin. When we are sleep-deprived, our skin takes on a pasty, puffy, and more wrinkled appearance," says Dr. Nicholas Perricone. During a good night of sleep (eight hours is ideal), the cells in your body do many amazing things, such as secrete growth hormone, which helps repair and rebuild muscle and bone and increase the production of proteins (needed for cell growth and to repair damage from stress and the sun). Another reason to get your *zzzs* is because that's when your skincare treatment products do what they're supposed to. "The skin's permeability also increases during sleep," says Dr. Perricone. "Thus, the benefits of topical antioxidants increases, giving new meaning to the term 'beauty sleep.'"

expert advice

SLEEPING TIPS FROM THE BEAUTY EXPERTS

- "Avoid any activities that have bright lights shining in your face, such as watching TV or working on the computer, at least an hour before going to sleep. Bright lights suppress the secretion of melatonin, a hormone that is a natural sleep inducer." —Dr. Perricone

- "If I follow this breathing technique, I'm generally asleep in five minutes: Breathe in at a count of four and breathe out at a count of four, in a way that's very rhythmic, so when you're switching from breathing in to breathing out, you're never holding your breath. This enables a steady flow of oxygen into the body and sends a message to the nervous system that you're in a relaxed state." —Sarah Kugelman

- "Keep the most boring book you can find on your nightstand and start reading it if you're having trouble falling asleep. I turn to car maintenance books—they put me right to sleep every time." —Leslie Blodgett

- "Count your blessings instead of sheep and think about all the things to be grateful about." —Hana Zalzal

- "I can't go to bed without smelling wonderful. At night, I do an Amazing Grace full-body scenting ritual. I take a bubble bath with the Amazing Grace Bath, Shampoo, and Shower Gel, moisturize with the body lotion, and then spray on the body oil. If I wake up in the middle of the night, all I have to do is smell my pajamas and I fall immediately back to sleep." —Cristina Carlino

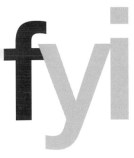

smoke ALARM

fyi

"When we inhale just one puff of a cigarette, over a trillion free radicals are produced in our lungs, which then trigger an inflammatory response that circulates throughout our body," says Dr. Perricone. Free radicals, the once healthy oxygen molecules that become overactive and unstable after losing an electron, attack DNA as they go about stealing electrons from the nearest stable and healthy cells in our body. "Inhaling tobacco causes a tremendous inflammatory response in all organs of the body—including the skin. Cigarette smoking depletes the skin of oxygen and vital nutrients including vitamin C, which is critical in keeping skin youthful, moist, and plumped up." Smoking can also lower estrogen levels in women; estrogen keeps the skin plump and increases collagen production. And let's not forget about the aging that occurs from the mechanical motions of smoking. "The puckering of the lips during smoking creates those smoker's lines," says Dr. Howard Sobel, dermatologist and founder of DDF. Moral of the story: *Don't smoke!* If you are a smoker, the best thing you can possibly do for your skin is to quit. Right now. "I've seen sets of twins in their fifties, one a smoker and one a nonsmoker. The smoker always looks twenty years older," says Dr. Perricone. Enough said.

fight free radicals!

Unfortunately, banning contact with cigarette smoke from your life doesn't remove all the danger of free radicals being introduced to the skin. Pollution, stress, and other environmental factors also produce free radicals. The good news is you can protect yourself with antioxidants, which act like kryptonite to those damaging free radicals. "Always wear an antioxidant-rich product underneath your sunscreen," says Dr. Brandt. "Look for ingredients such as green tea, grapeseed, and white tea—they act like a sponge, sucking up any free radicals before they interact with the skin."

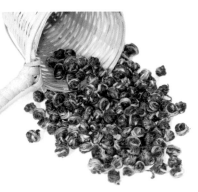

BEAUTY secret

"In the summer when my skin is
dry or sunburned, I apply olive oil
to it. It's a trick I learned from my
Spanish aunt."

—Dany Sanz

SUN SMARTS

Photoaging, the technical term used to describe sun damage, can take years to show up on our skin. But every time you expose yourself to the sun sans protection, the skin loses the ability to repair itself, collagen and elastin become damaged, and that damage accumulates. Skin becomes saggy, wrinkled, and leathery, and fails to spring back. And forget about throwing pricey skin care at the problem. "I've seen so many women try to undo the damage with expensive skin-care products, but who still leave their skin unprotected from the sun during the day," says Dr. Brandt. "They're just going in circles!" In other words, you have two options if you want to hold on to a healthy, young complexion: Either use sun protection, or stay out of the sun entirely!

sun care FAQs

Q: What's the difference between UVA and UVB rays?

a: UVB and UVA are the invisible ultraviolet rays emitted from the sun. UVA rays are known as the aging rays because they penetrate the skin more deeply and cause wrinkles. UVA rays can go through windows and through your clothing, so you're always in danger of exposure. They can also crack and shrink the collagen and elastin in our skin. The destruction of collagen (which makes up 75 percent of our skin) and elastin (a protein in connective tissue that allows the skin to resume its shape after stretching or contracting) leads to the loss of skin's strength and elasticity, thus causing wrinkles and sagging, leathery skin. And if aged skin wasn't bad enough, studies show that UVA exacerbates UVB's carcinogenic effects and may induce some skin cancers, including melanomas. UVB, the burn ray, affects the epidermis (the outer layer of skin) and is the main cause of skin cancer. Melanoma, the deadliest form of skin cancer, kills about 8,000 people each year. UVA rays stimulate the melanocyte cells (located in the bottom layer of the skin) to produce the brown pigment melanin, aka a suntan. So the next time you compliment someone's post-Caribbean vacation glow, keep in mind their suntan is actually a sign that their skin's been injured.

Q: What's the difference between sunscreen and sunblock?

a: Sunscreen is classified as chemical, while sunblock is physical. Sunscreens absorb and reflect the ultraviolet radiation, while sunblock physically blocks both the UVA and UVB radiation from the skin. Sunblock is made of either titanium oxide or zinc oxide. Some common active ingredients in sunscreens include aminobenzoic acid (PABA), avobenzone, oxybenzone, homosalate, cinoxate, and octyl salicylate. Sunscreen takes about twenty to thirty minutes to really penetrate the skin, which is why you need to apply it at least half an hour before sun exposure.

Q: How much sunscreen should I be using?

a: Always be generous when applying sunscreen. You should see a film at first wherever you apply it, before it sinks into skin. Always apply at least one ounce, about the amount in a shot glass, to cover all exposed parts of the body. Always store sunscreen in a cool, dry place, and it should remain stable and at its original strength for almost three years. But the truth is a bottle of sunscreen *shouldn't* last that long. "If you have sunscreen left over from a year ago, you're not using enough!" says Dr. Brandt.

Q: How often should I reapply?

a: The American Academy of Dermatology says to reapply every two hours, even on cloudy days. But if you're doing any activities that involve sweating or swimming, you should be reapplying more often. "There are a number of mechanical actions that remove sunscreen. These include swimming, drying off with a towel, and perspiring," says Dr. Perricone.

Q: What areas on my face and body should I be hyperaware of protecting with sunscreen?

a: "A lot of people neglect their chest, neck, and décolletage," says Dr. Murad. "That's an important area to cover because the skin here is very thin and there's no direct muscle that it attaches to." Another area you want to slather with SPF is the backs of your hands. They're one of the first spots on the body to show aging. "There's not much a dermatologist or a plastic surgeon can do for you once you've damaged the skin on your hands," says Peter Thomas Roth.

expert advice

HOW TO OUTSMART THE SUN'S HARMFUL RAYS

- "I take the window seat on airplanes just so I have control over the shade—making sure it's always down to block the sun. I always walk on the shady side of the street and my car has dark-tinted windows." —Dr. Fredric Brandt

- "Wear a shirt or a surfer's rash guard over your bikini, even if you're wearing sunscreen." —Peter Thomas Roth

- "I always keep a big sun hat in my car just in case I get a flat tire in the middle of the day and have to wait outside for help." —Leslie Blodgett

words **of wisdom**

"I really believe the number one secret to looking and feeling young is to find every opportunity to laugh. Having your face frozen in stress and frowns will instantly age you. People who laugh a lot have this spark about them and this glimmer in their eye that can't be replaced—not even with makeup!"

—Leslie Blodgett

STRESSING OUT

Stress is a part of everyday life. From traffic jams and deadlines to breakups and problems at work, we all feel stressed out sometimes. Stress can manifest itself by giving us tense muscles, headaches, and anxiety, but you may not realize the toll it takes on the complexion. "Stress increases oil production on the skin, which is why we break out sometimes when we get stressed," explains Skyn Iceland founder Sarah Kugelman. "It also impairs the lipid barrier function, so when you're stressed, skin loses that healthy, youthful glow." Stress can also make you look much older than you are. "Stress creates internal inflammation, which has been linked to premature aging," says Kugelman. Since avoiding stress altogether isn't realistic, how you deal with it can make all the difference in your life—and skin.

the top 5 ways to de-stress

1 Exercise on a regular basis—it helps fight stress and depression, not to mention love handles. Exercise doesn't have to mean getting on the treadmill again. Go outside for a fifteen-minute walk during lunch, or try yoga, Pilates, or a dance class.

2 Allow yourself more time to get places than you think you'll need, especially if it's an important meeting or interview. Nothing's more stressful than being late.

3 Make time to talk to your friends. Even if it's just for ten minutes, a phone call to your favorite person can help.

4 Make a de-stress playlist of your favorite calming songs on your iPod and listen to it whenever you feel like you want to scream.

5 Treat yourself to a massage or have a spa day at home. It can be as simple as putting on a mask and relaxing. Or create a steam room in the bathroom by letting the hot water run before a shower and sitting in there for five to ten minutes.

expert advice
STRESS-BUSTING TIPS FROM THE PROS

- "Meditation and breathing techniques don't cost a dime and you can do them anywhere, anytime." —Sarah Kugelman

- "To fight stress throughout the day, I get up from my workspace and stretch. First, I lean forward and touch my palms to the floor, while I focus on constricting my stomach muscles. I hold this for a minute, and then I bend my knees lightly as I roll into the upright position and reach my hands up toward the ceiling."—Ole Henriksen

- "I take a warm bath with pure lavender oil and have a cup of organic chamomile tea." —Carol Shaw

- "Eliminate toxic people from your environment." —Karen Behnke

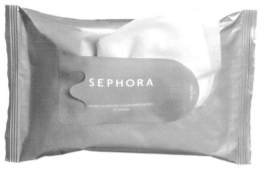

skin SMARTS

SKYN ICELAND ICELANDIC RELIEF EYE CREAM WITH BIOSPHERIC COMPLEX

This light-as-air eye cream delivers major impact to the stressed-out eye area. Rice peptides help counteract the aging effects of stress, optical diffusers soften fine lines and brighten the eye area, vitamin K increases circulation to lighten dark circles, and Icelandic kelp helps fight inflammation.

KINERASE INTENSIVE EYE CREAM

Your eyes are one of the first areas to show age. Keep them guessing yours with this potent eye cream. It contains 0.125 percent Kinetin, the highest level of this antiaging ingredient available in any product.

SEPHORA BRAND MAKEUP REMOVING WIPES

Going to sleep with your makeup on is a big beauty no-no. Make the washing-up process less painful with these soft facial cleansing cloths saturated with FACE Fluid Makeup Remover. Cleanses and eliminates all types of makeup, even long-wearing, from the face, eyes, and lips without an oily residue.

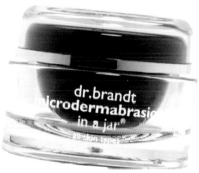

DR. BRANDT MICRODERMABRASION

Dr. Brandt brings the ever-popular in-office procedure to our homes with this jar of diamond-shaped magnesium oxide crystals. After exfoliation, skin is left glowing, healthy, and smooth as a baby's bottom.

PTR BOTANICAL BUFFING BEADS

We have yet to meet someone who hasn't fallen for this award-winning blue bottle. The secret sauce, a blend of ultrafine jojoba beads and botanical nutrients, exfoliates dead surface skin cells, opens clogged pores, and emulsifies the sebum that contributes to blackheads and whiteheads.

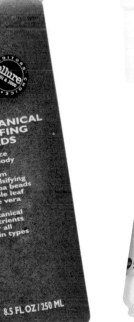

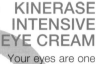

BLISS SLEEPING PEEL

Get your beauty sleep with this supercharged skin-rejuvenating serum. This amino-acid exfoliant works like a dream as it sloughs off dry skin, minimizes pores, and fades fine lines and dark spots while you're getting your *zzz*s.

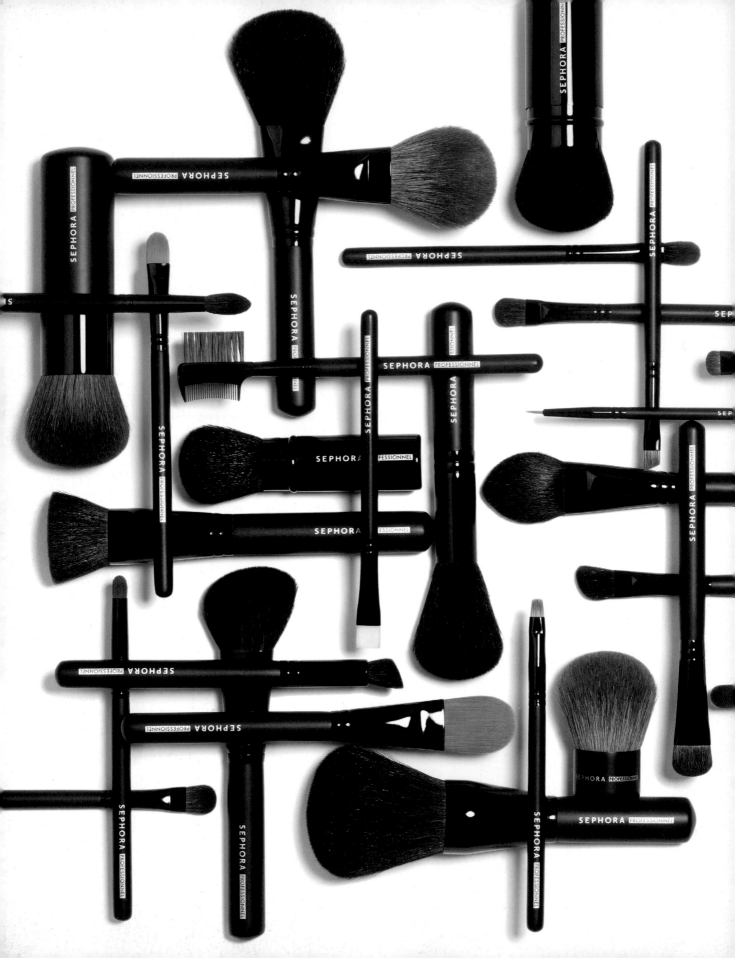

tools of attraction

"Makeup brushes bring makeup to life," says Ross Burton of Lancôme. Indeed, without the right brush to apply your blush, it's just a square of pretty pink powder sitting in a compact. Not only do makeup brushes provide a professional and more natural-looking finish on your face, but they'll also save you time and money in the long run. Brushes pick up and distribute product without absorbing it—hence making your makeup last a lot longer than if you were using only your fingers all the time. Unfortunately, though, most brushes and tools don't come with instruction manuals. We've decoded the whos, whats, and whys of all the mysterious looking beauty tools, including a few household objects. We'll bet you'll never look at a spoon the same way again.

concealer brush

What it's for: Applying any cream product, including concealer, eye primer, and eye cream. The thin tapered top is perfect for concealing dark circles in the corner of eyes, the entire eyelid, or the area around the nose.

Why it works: The tapered head fits into the contours of the face, in corner of eyes, and right under the lash line. The synthetic fibers won't absorb any product, so it will save you time and money.

How to use it: Load the brush tip with concealer, dab onto area to be covered, and feather edges until blended.

foundation brush

What it's for: Applying foundation or moisturizer or masks.

Why it works: It won't absorb oils or product and it's much more hygienic to use than your fingers. The thin, oval flower tip accesses all the recessed and contoured areas of the face.

How to use it: Start at the center of the face and blend down and out in the direction of the natural hairs, blending past the jawline so there's no line of demarcation.

Pro tip: Use it to mix moisturizer into your foundation to make the formula more sheer. Use it with a cream blush to really melt it into your skin. It's also a perfect eraser if you've made too many mistakes or applied too much product.

complexion brush

What it's for: Setting your foundation with powder and toning down shine.

Why it works: Tapered head and chiseled cut allows for even distribution of pressed, loose, or translucent powder, blush, and bronzer. Hand-shaped hairs and domed top fit beautifully into contours of face and distributes color evenly.

How to use it: Dip brush into powder and gently tap brush onto a tissue to eliminate excess. Apply all over face or wherever needed with a gentle sweeping motion.

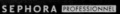

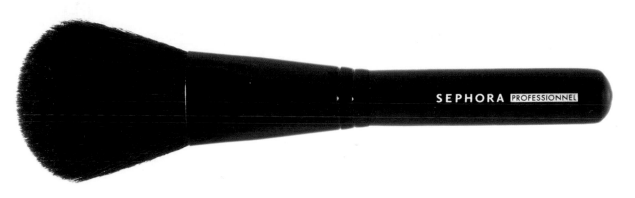

powder brush

What it's for: Applying loose or pressed powder after your foundation to extend the wear of your makeup.

Why it works: Goat hair gives you more control of where you're placing product and it's perfect for blending on neck and décolletage. The short handle makes it easy to use, even for novices.

How to use it: Focus on center of face—make sure it's smooth and even, because that's the surface that people see. Focus on forehead, nose, chin, and jawline.

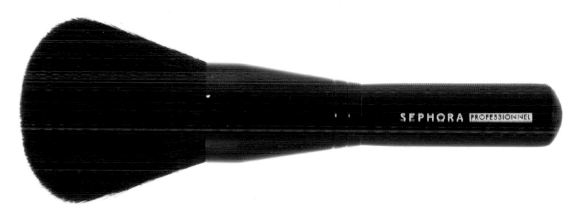

rounded powder brush

What it's for: Applying pressed powder, loose powder, bronzer, and for contouring. Powdering all over—shoulders and décolletage.

Why it works: The expansive head allows for all-over application. It fits seamlessly into contours and blends with ease.

How to use it: Dip into powder and tap excess product off into a tissue or you can get buildup, which makes for a blotchy complexion.

retractable powder brush

What it's for: This one is multipurpose and amazing for traveling.

Why it works: The lightweight metal encasing is adjustable, so you can lower for full coverage or bring it up for more concentration of pigment (ideal for eye shadow). Also use it with mineral makeup.

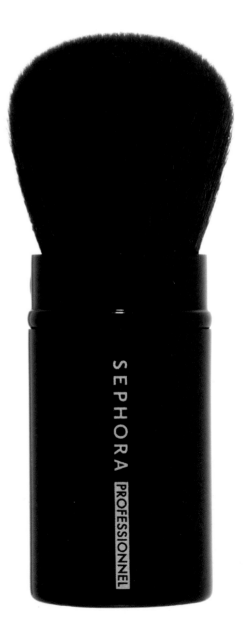

kabuki brush

What it's for: Leaving an airbrushed finish when applying mineral makeup, loose powder, and bronzer.

Why it works: The nub end fits perfectly into the palm of your hand. Dense bristles allow for full coverage and more control.

How to use it: Dip brush into powder or mineral makeup and gently tap the brush onto a tissue or lid to eliminate excess. Apply all over the face or where needed with a gentle, circular buffing motion.

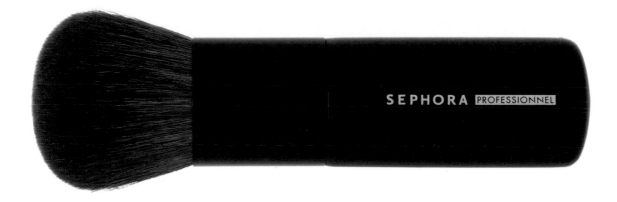

bronzer brush

What it's for: Applying bronzer onto cheeks, forehead, chin, and shoulders for a realistic golden glow.

Why it works: The rounded, tapered end fits perfectly into the cheekbones. The soft goat hair blends beautifully.

How to use it: Dip brush into powder and tap off excess. Use a circular, buffing motion to glide brush over skin, going right into contours of cheeks. Apply between orbital bone and jawbone and blend down. It can also be used to apply translucent powder using same method for added coverage.

angled blush brush

What it's for: Precisely defining cheekbones with blush, bronzer, or contour color

Why it works: The angled shape picks up on the contours of your face with strategically placed slanted natural hairs allowing you to apply color exactly where you want it. It fills in contours so your cheekbones will really pop.

How to use it: The slanted hairs pick up more product, so make sure to tap off excess before applying. Find your cheekbone and with short strokes, brush up at an angle toward your ears.

rounded blush brush

What it's for: Highlighting the orbital bone (area around the eye), applying blush or bronzer; chiseled bristles give even distribution.

Why it works: The longer bristles and rounded head allow for a more evenly dispersed application and create a natural-looking glow.

How to use it: On orbital bone, dust a pink or white highlighting powder on the C area around the eyes. On cheeks, smile and place the blush onto apples of cheeks to brighten up the entire face.

Pro Tip: To find natural blush color, swipe shades of blush onto the palms of hands and see what complements the natural coloring there.

flat blush brush

What it's for: Great for giving the entire face a sculpted look, and for a deeper hit of blush.

Why it works: Flat, tapered point gives you more concentration of color.

How to use it: Line up the point of the brush on the cheekbone, and sweep along the bone. To sculpt the face, dip the brush into a light bisque shade and use the pointed edge to outline the hairline and the area below the jawline. Use fingers to blend.

contour blush brush

What it's for: Creating perfectly contoured cheeks.

Why it works: The secret is in the flat end of this brush, which allows you to apply plenty of color right where you want it, for professionally sculpted cheeks.

How to use it: Dip the brush into a contour color (usually a shade or two darker than your skin tone), then tap off excess product. Suck in cheeks and follow line directly underneath the cheekbone. Start near the hairline and bring the product in—don't start from center of face, as you will deliver too much product at first.

brow brush

What it's for: Applying brow wax, powder, gel, or pencil.

Why it works: The thickness allows for precision to create the shape brow you desire. Bristles are synthetic and wax-friendly.

How to use it: Start where hair is thickest for a natural look. Using short strokes, mimic the hair on your brows, filling in only where you need color. If you don't have a lot of hair, use wax. End at the angle of where the eye ends.

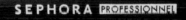

brow and lash comb

What it's for: Eyebrow and eyelash grooming.

Why it works: The plastic side is used to clean up mascara and to rid lashes of clumping; the brush side to blend in brow color.

How to use it: After mascara application, comb the plastic bristles through lashes from roots to ends. Dip brush side in brow color and brush through brows, or use it to blend in pencil.

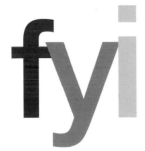

fyi

Natural bristles (sable, pony, squirrel, and goat hairs) are softer and more porous so they hold on to pigment extremely well.

VS **Synthetic bristles** are more suitable for applying cream and liquid products, as they prevent streaking.

rounded smudge brush

What it's for: Applying dark, intense color to the eyelids, or lining the eye with a thick line of color. It's also great for applying color to the creases.

Why it works: Domed tip fits perfectly into crease—hairs are dense so there's more color pickup. It can also be used underneath the eye as an eyeliner brush.

How to use it: Apply crease color with eye open initially until you get used to it, then you can do it with eyes closed. Mark the placement first with a dab of color and then blend.

rounded crease brush

What it's for: Accentuating crease.

Why it works: The thin shape and tapered end are great for precision and fit perfectly in crease.

How to use it: Apply color with eye opened, using short strokes and making sure it blends. A must-have if you're just learning how to apply shadow.

smudge brush

What it's for: Creating a sexy, sultry, smoky-eye look.

Why it works: The shorter bristles give you more precision and do exactly as promised— soften and smudge lines. Use small strokes instead of swiping. Small enough to use over eyelid. Stay close to lashline, apply evenly, and smudge it out.

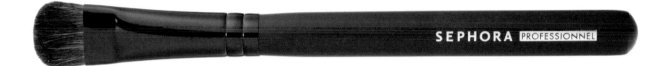

angled eyeliner brush

What it's for: Applying liquid, cream, and powder liner.

Why it works: The tapered point fits perfectly against the eyelid, allowing you to apply a superthin line for a natural look.

How to use it: Dip it into the liner, close the eyelid you're working on and gently flick it up and out at the end for a dramatic cat-eye look.

all-over eye shadow brush

What it's for: Applying base color all over the lid.

Why it works: The wide, expansive head fits into the entire lid in just a couple strokes. Bristles are condensed, which allows products to go right where you need it. Hairs are evenly distributed so you get an even distribution of color.

How to use it: Dip brush into powder, tap off excess product, and press it into the entire lid, from lashline to brows.

angled shadow brush

What it's for: Adding color to contour, in the crease or right underneath the brow bone.

Why it works: The angle fits directly into the crease and perfectly under the orbital bone.

How to use it: To use in crease, turn it so the pointy part is in the crease and the brush will guide you for perfect product placement. To use under brows, dip into a shimmery pink or white shadow and turn brush so the pointy part is directly under the arch.

SEPHORA PROFESSIONNEL

small synthetic eye shadow brush

What it's for: Applying cream eye shadow, eye primer, eye cream.

Why it works: You won't waste cream products—synthetic doesn't absorb.

How to use it: Go into the crease with shadow and use the flat tip with eye shadow. Also use it to apply highlighter right into brow bone with short strokes.

SEPHORA PROFESSIONNEL

sponge tip shadow applicator

What it's for: Blending.

Why it works: Latex foam tip, so it's very durable.

How to use it: Apply eyeliner with it—or dip into shadow to apply a smoky eye. Blends pencil perfectly—great for those who don't have a steady hand when applying liner.

SEPHORA PROFESSIONNEL

blending eye brush

What it's for: Blending.

Why it works: Bristles are wider to grab color and blend it all together.

How to use it: After applying color, blend it out with this brush—this is the last brush you should use on lids. It will blend out any imperfections. Apply over shadow you've already applied. When you press, bristles spread out. The colors should blend into each other—there should never be any harsh lines.

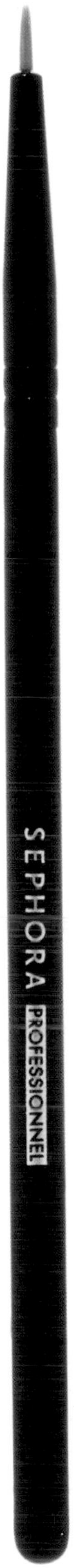

pointed eyeliner brush

What it's for: Applying liquid liner.

Why it works: The fine point allows you to do a superthin or thick line. Short handles make it easy to use. Bristles fit perfectly right into lashline. Pointed and tapered for the thinnest line possible, this brush is made with synthetic fibers for precise application. It's perfect for lining upper and lower lashlines with cream-based liners, or your favorite eye shadow.

How to use it: Always start thin and you can build on the line—it's much harder to take away. Only a little pressure is needed—the brush does all the work.

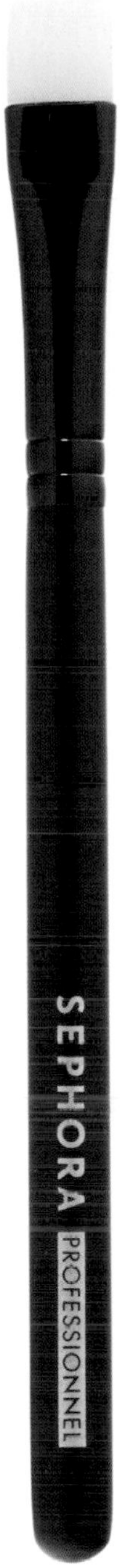

SEPHORA PROFESSIONNEL

flat eyeliner brush

What it's for: Applying eyeliner—cream, liquid, or powder.

Why it works: The synthetic bristles hold any formulation while you can see the color you're applying.

How to use it: Dip into color, then go right into the lashline with the tip of the brush.

SEPHORA PROFESSIONNEL

BEAUTY tip

Always tap excess powder off your brush before applying color.

lip brush

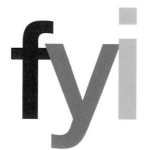

What it's for: A precise and professional-looking lipstick and lip gloss application.

Why it works: The tug-proof bristles are extra-precise, allowing you to layer lipstick and lip gloss to achieve your desired degree of fullness.

How to use it: Dip into lipstick or gloss and blend in color and contour lips with short strokes. Use your finger to smudge it in for a natural, just-bitten look.

toothbrush

What it's for: Exfoliating lips, brushing eyebrow hairs into place, taming fly-aways.

How to use it: On lips, gently rub on lips that have a lip balm or an exfoliating lip product on them. To tame fly-aways, spritz it with hairspray and comb the frazzled strands.

spoon

What it's for: De-puffing eyelids and to protect eye makeup from stray mascara.

How to use it: For eyelids: Put the spoon in the freezer for about thirty minutes. Place it, rounded side down, on top of closed lids for about ten minutes. To protect eye makeup: Place spoon, convex side down, over lid before applying mascara.

fyi

Smaller brushes are best for detailed precision work (i.e., covering blemishes, blood vessels, and dark circles). The shorter hairs offer better control in the more contoured areas of the face.

beauty school:
how to clean your brushes

1 Remove excess color from the brush with a tissue.

2 Run brush under water just long enough to dampen the hairs.

3 Place a small amount of gentle shampoo onto the palm of your hand and swirl the dampened brush in your palm for a few moments.

4 Place the brush under warm running water with brush hairs facing down. Gently squeeze the hairs until the water runs clear.

5 Squeeze the clean brush hairs to remove any excess water.

6 Avoid soaking the brush or allowing too much water to run into the ferrule (the barrel of the brush), which will break down the glue and loosen the hairs of the brush.

7 Lay brushes flat, or with bristles at a slight downward angle, on a paper or cotton towel to dry overnight.

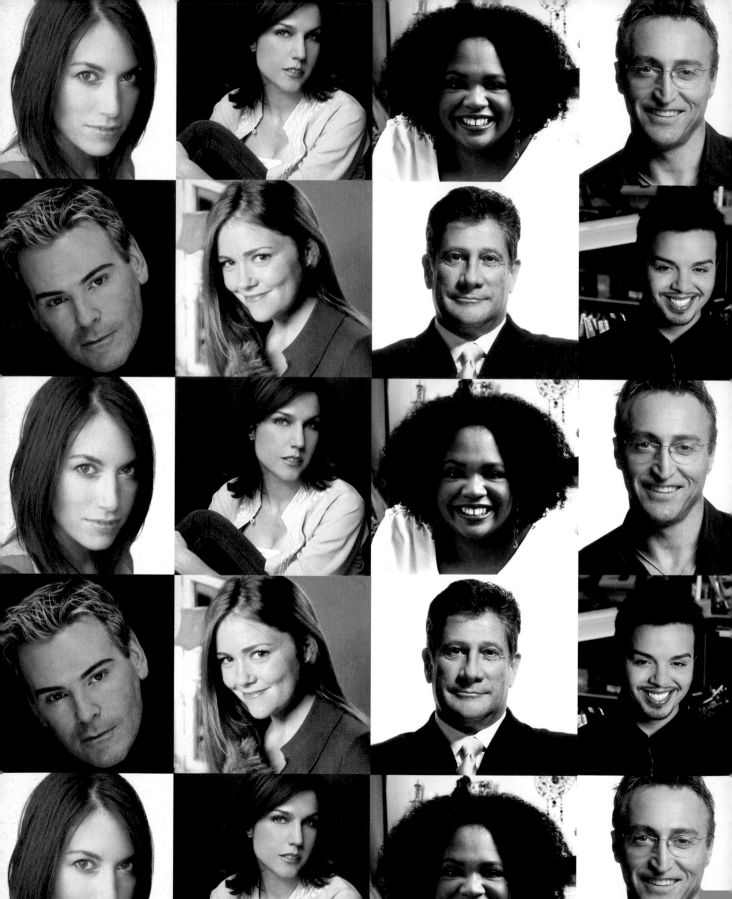

meet the masters

We'd like to introduce you to the personalities behind your favorite brands. Our masters spend each day deep in the beauty trenches, discovering new ways to look and feel exceptional. In this chapter, you'll get an exclusive look into the private lives of Sephora's top beauty gurus, including Dr. Perricone, Oscar Blandi, Wende Zomnir, Sue Devitt, Maureen Kelly, Ole Henriksen, Leslie Blodgett, Lisa Price, Davis Factor, Jerrod Blandino, Vincent Longo, and Cristina Bartolucci. There's a lot to learn from these passionate men and women behind the curtain, including what it truly means to be beautiful.

BEAUTY DIARY: GILBERT SOLIZ

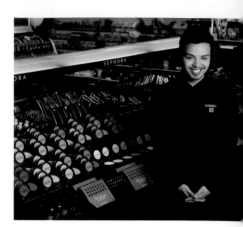

Spend a beauty-filled day with Sephora Pro Beauty Team artist Gilbert Soliz at the Glendale, California, Sephora store.

11 am

I arrive at Glendale, one of the biggest malls in Los Angeles. Our store boasts some of the highest amounts of traffic in any Sephora location in Southern California! I work mid-shifts, so my day starts a bit later. The first thing we do is gather around and touch base with the DIC (director in charge) to gear up for another big day in our beauty wonderland.

11:15 am

Each day, I select a "passion item" I want to share with clients. This week, it's Dior Show Mascara. This product literally does it all for the lashes. It doesn't smear or smudge, and it curls while it volumizes—it's truly amazing. Whenever I apply it on clients, they immediately run to the register with it.

11:30 am

A young client comes to me with skin concerns. We have a lot of teenagers in the mall looking for ways to clear up their acne. I understand that this can be a very personal concern for some people. I direct my client to the Murad Acne Complex Starter Kit, which is a full regimen complete with a bacteria-fighting cleanser, exfoliator, treatment, and lotion. Whenever my clients buy the kit, nine times out of ten, they come back and buy the full-size products.

noon

A thirtysomething client walks in search of a new look, and we walk around the store together choosing products that speak to her. I talk the client through every step as I put the makeup on her, and I jot down all the products and apply the same colors to the face chart, which always ends up looking like a piece of art. My client ends up buying a pink glittery lipstick and the Diamond Shadow from Make Up For Ever. She's really excited when she finds out she can take the face chart home.

12:30 pm

I start talking to a mature client who tells me she's never liked foundation because she's always felt like it was too heavy on her face. I sit her down and show her my stippling technique with Nars Balance Foundation in Budapest. I start with a pea-sized amount of foundation, and instead of applying it with a wiping motion, it's more of a bouncing motion with the sponge. I apply only on the areas that need coverage. The effect is a really natural, yet flawless, finish. She's shocked about how much it brightened and lifted her face.

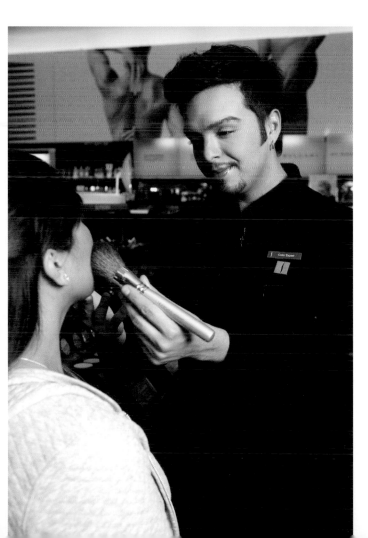

4:00 pm

I go to my designated zone to touch up my AOP (Area of Pride). At the moment I'm in love with Nars Blush in Luster, which is really more of a complexion booster than a blush. It's a golden beige that gives the skin this gorgeous veil of luminosity. I'm also loving Nars Night Rider eye shadow, this really cool plum shade with white and silver chunks in it.

5 pm

I head backstage (the office and stockroom area) and sit down with the other beauty experts to talk about any makeup tricks and ideas I've learned recently. Being part of the Sephora Pro Team, I'm exposed to all the trends at the New York and Los Angeles fashion weeks, and I like to bring it back and show the rest of the cast so they can try them too. Today I tell them about the "moved matte" finish I learned backstage at LA Fashion Week. It's a really natural-looking finish you get by using a powder puff and translucent powder to set different areas of the face. The goal is to eliminate shine on the chin, forehead, and right below the cheekbones, while leaving the rest of the face untouched with powder so it remains dewy and gives skin a natural finish. I love to see them share these tips, tricks, and beauty looks with our clients.

MASTER STASHES: DR. PERRICONE

Renowned dermatologist Dr. Nicholas Perricone, who believes you are what you eat, opens up the door of his refrigerator to reveal antioxidant, protein-rich foods that make your skin glow and your mind sharp.

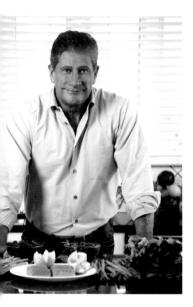

A very low-grade form of inflammation goes on in the body every day—this is something we can't see or feel—but it causes damages to organ systems and accelerates the aging process. This increases our risk of age-related diseases as well as wrinkled, sagging skin. I've found that foods are extremely important in terms of fighting inflammation in the body, so over a period of ten years I developed the anti-inflammatory diet. The principles are fairly simple: Choose foods that are rich in antioxidants and healthy fats like the omegas 3, 6, and 9, found in foods such as salmon and olive oil. The anti-inflammatory diet contains the foods that your grandmother recommended: simple, natural, and wholesome. Reasonable amounts of a wide variety of natural foods: fresh fish and poultry or tofu, brightly colored fresh fruits and vegetables. Look for the rainbow foods—the more colors you see means the more antioxidant and anti-inflammatory activity.

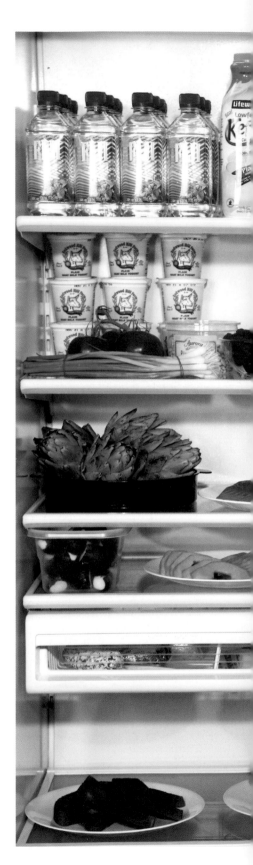

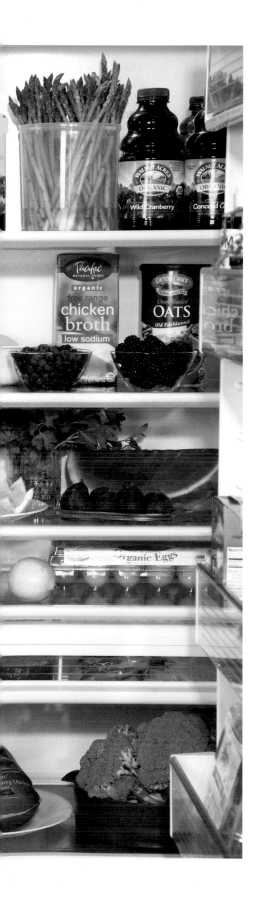

in dr. perricone's fridge

KEFIR This is a probiotic, cultured milk, containing very friendly bacteria. It's also a good source of calcium and protein. I put a healthy handful of raspberries, blueberries, and pomegranate extract in the blender, and then add plain, unsweetened kefir. It makes a really delicious drink that tastes like a berry milkshake.

FIJI NATURAL SPRING WATER Water is important—if you do not drink water, your organs and cells cannot function. You don't have to overdo it, but if you don't drink water, you cannot metabolize fat, nor can you flush wastes out of the cells. A dehydrated body provokes the development of aging, inflammatory compounds. Water has great anti-inflammatory properties and will help your skin to be radiant, soft, and supple.

You can also eat fruits such as cantaloupe, which contain a lot of natural moisture as well as skin-beautifying vitamins, nutrients, and antioxidants. Whenever possible, choose pure spring water such as Poland Spring or FIJI. Tap water can have impurities, such as chlorine, that aren't the best for us. FIJI water also contains silica, an essential mineral, that can help strengthen bones, connective tissue, teeth, skin, hair, and nails.

ORGANIC CHICKEN Choose organic free-range chicken, free of antibiotics and hormones. Chicken (minus the skin) is low in saturated fat and a great source of protein. I like to prepare it in a stir-fry, or roasted, baked, or broiled.

BROCCOLI One of my favorite vegetables! A lot of great research shows that broccoli inhibits cancer because it contains active chemicals called indole-3-carbinol, also found in Brussels sprouts and cauliflower.

ASPARAGUS High in antioxidants, fiber, and potassium! A great food. Asparagus also contains a unique type of carbohydrate called inulin that we don't digest, but the health-promoting friendly bacteria in our large intestine, such as bifidobacteria and lactobacilli, do. Asparagus is cardio-protective and prevents birth defects thanks to its high levels of folate. It also acts as a natural diuretic.

WILD ALASKAN SALMON

I eat a lot of fish! Wild salmon and other coldwater fish (sardines, herring, trout) are great sources of protein, which is necessary to maintain and repair the body—including the skin on a cellular level. Protein cannot be stored in our bodies. For optimum health and cellular repair, we need to have a good source of quality protein at each meal. Coldwater fish is also high in anti-inflammatory omega 3 essential fatty acids, which keep skin radiant, supple, and wrinkle-free; moods upbeat; and brain functioning at optimal levels. Wild salmon's bright pink or deep red color owes its pigment to the presence of astaxanthin, a super powerful carotenoid antioxidant with potent anti-inflammatory properties. Wild Alaskan salmon is my favorite because it is low in toxins, high in protein and essential fats—and it is also a very sustainable resource that the planet provides for us.

CHICKEN BROTH I use organic, free-range chicken broth as a base for soups and for cooking in general. For extra flavor, I add chicken broth to the bottom of the pan when I roast a chicken to keep the chicken moist and flavorful.

SLOW-COOKED OATS Slow-cooked oats are not rapidly absorbed by the bloodstream, preventing a rapid rise in blood sugar. Instant oats are not recommended, as they are rapidly absorbed, converting to sugar in the body, raising levels of blood sugar and insulin, causing inflammation.

JUICE In general, juices are not recommended because they rapidly convert to sugar in the bloodstream, causing inflammation and accelerating aging, wrinkles, weight gain, etc. However some juices can be enjoyed, such as pomegranate and unsweetened cranberry, as they are lower on the glycemic index.

GOAT'S MILK YOGURT Yogurt is probiotic and very high in protein. Goat milk's ease of digestibility is due to the fact that it has smaller fat particles than those found in cow's milk. It is also a good source of calcium, protein, phosphorous, vitamin B12, and potassium.

BLUEBERRIES, RASPBERRIES, AND BLACKBERRIES I call these the "magic berries." All three are high in antioxidants, but blueberries in particular are very powerful, because they contain powerful phytochemical antioxidants such as the anthocyanins. These phytochemicals speed up neural communications and prevent cell death and the loss of nerve growth factors. Blueberries also give the brain a greater ability to release dopamine, an energizing, stimulatory neurotransmitter. Blueberries also protect us from the loss of dopamine cells that is normally seen with aging. By increasing brain energy production and maintaining youthful brain function, dopamine exerts an extremely important anti-aging effect. Since dopamine decreases with age, blueberries become even more important as we get older.

AVOCADO For years, many people avoided avocados because they are high in fat. However, most of the fat in an avocado is monounsaturated, the kind that protects against heart disease and certain cancers. Monounsaturated fat is burned more efficiently after exercise than saturated fat, a fact that may significantly contribute to long-term weight loss. Avocados also contain omega 3 fatty acids, important for healthy skin and brain functioning and facilitating weight loss. Omega 3s are also cardio-protective and reduce inflammation.

FRESH FIGS Figs are not only delicious, they are very high in antioxidants. I enjoy them fresh and raw. Figs are an excellent source of calcium and potassium, a mineral that helps to control blood pressure.

WATERMELON Another mainstay. Watermelon is a great fruit high in important anti-aging antioxidants, including vitamins C and A. Watermelon is also a highly concentrated source of the carotenoid lycopene, which has powerful anticancer properties. Like cantaloupe, watermelon is also refreshing and hydrating.

ARTICHOKE They're loaded with antioxidants! Specifically, artichokes contain antioxidants that protect the liver, such as silymarin. Since ancient times, the artichoke has been used for liver and gallbladder conditions, "cleansing" the blood as well as the bladder. Artichokes are also very high in fiber, potassium, calcium, iron, phosphorus, and other trace elements important for a balanced system. I enjoy artichokes trimmed, steamed, and then lightly dressed with fresh minced garlic, lemon juice, and extra-virgin olive oil.

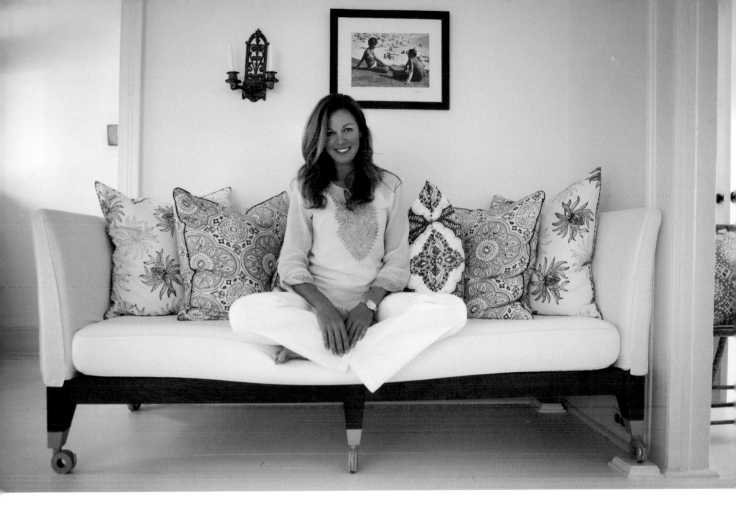

HOW TO THROW A SPA DAY: SUE DEVITT

How makeup artist and creator of microquatic spa products Sue Devitt treats her gals to a day of pampering.

I am extremely fortunate to have a very close group of girlfriends (my "pretty posse") who have become my personal brand sounding board of directors. They make themselves available to me within a moment's notice, twenty-four hours a day, eight days a week, for important and immediate feedback on beauty-related issues. They are always there for me and I adore each and every one of them. Every once in a while I host a spa day at my house to pamper them. Everyone leaves relaxed, happy, and rejuvenated. Here's how you can do the same for your "pretty posse."

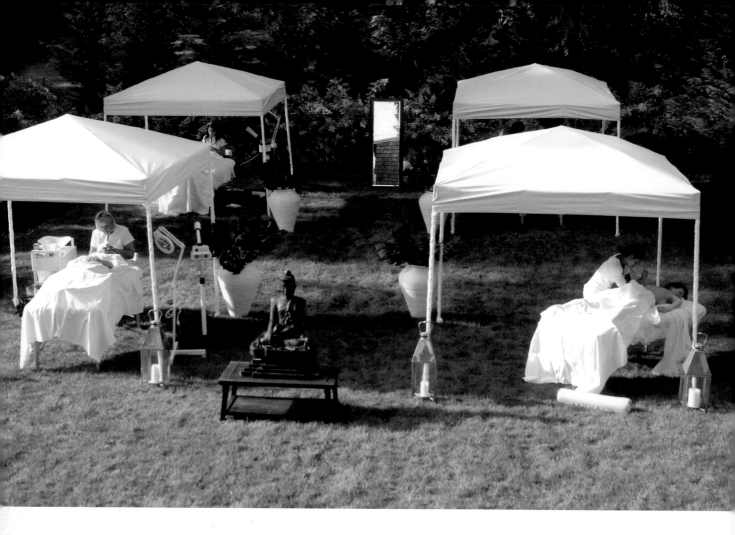

mi casa, su spa

For my spa day, I transform my yard into an elegant, peaceful, tranquil luxury spa lounge. This is what you'll need to do the same:

- Plush throws to drape over the couches and chairs. It gives the whole space a beautiful, ethereal feel.
- Scented candles scattered throughout the area you'll be in.
- Spa robes for your guests to change into.
- Soothing spa music playing in the background to create the right atmosphere.
- Plush pillows scattered everywhere for guests to lounge on.

create a spa menu

Assign each girlfriend a different spa treatment. Create a menu with fun names describing each service. (For example: "It's a wrap": a detoxifying facial with a marine mud mask.)

serve drinks with a spa twist

Create a menu of cocktails with relaxing names and refreshing ingredients. This is what I served at my spa day:

The Cool Cucumber: Lime, cucumber, mint, soda, a dash of rosewater, and a dash of vodka

The Anti-Ager: Champagne with a dash of pomegranate liqueur

The Au Naturel: Chilled unfiltered sake

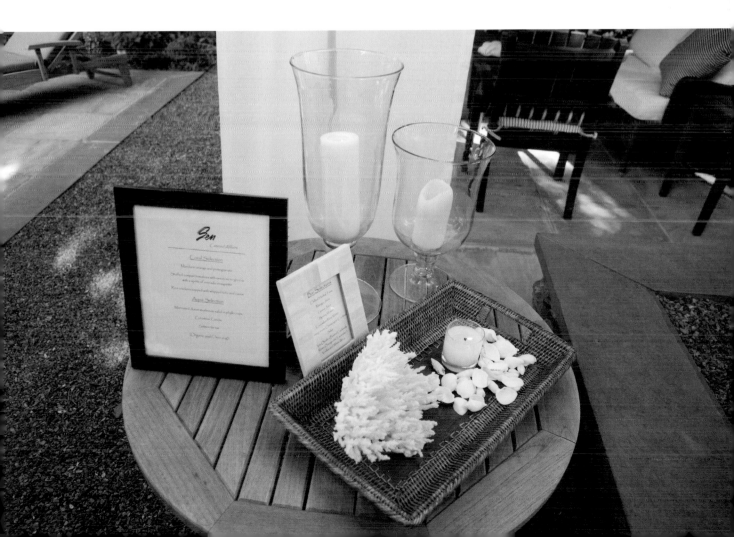

BEAUTY DIARY: LESLIE BLODGETT

A day at the office for Leslie Blodgett, CEO of Bare Escentuals, is anything but typical.

6:30 am alarm

Time to wake up!

7:15 am

Breakfast with my son, Trent. We literally spend five minutes together. I do some form of cardio if I'm inside.

8:30 am

On my way in to the office; I love my CDs and the drive over the Golden Gate Bridge.

9 am-ish

Jolt of caffeine when I get in. Caffeine is mood-altering for me. It makes me so happy, and then I'm ready for my run—around the office—shouting hellos to anyone who will listen. This is where I notice cute outfits, great eye shadow combos (you better be wearing eye makeup in this office!). I love when the gals get creative. It isn't unusual for me to take off my shoes so I can move faster. I love heels, but they're made for standing, not running.

9:45 am

Ahhhh, a product development meeting. The conference room is all set up with boards, plates of bareMinerals to review, a list of potential shade names, and package designs. This meeting is my favorite—great team, very creative energy—but sometimes we have way too much fun, thus the occasionally bizarre ideas we come up with. We like our products to work, heal the skin, and be fun at the same time. I need to see color combos on dozens of colleagues to make sure they work on several skin tones. I also like to hear as much customer feedback as possible on products in test. If they aren't just right, we're back to work until they are.

11:30 am

Run to the visual merchandising area to see what they have displayed on the wall—signage, photography. Run into the sales team office to see if all of our initiatives with our Sephora team are on track.

12:30 pm

Lunch—not much—soup, chicken breast, leftovers of whatever I had for dinner the night before.

1:15 pm

Run to Staci, our senior vice president, to see if she likes my new ideas. My big inspirations come at night and on weekends when I'm away from the office. Bare Escentuals Buxom Lips is an example. I had been trying to think of a word that really suggests big, full, and healthy— Jayne Mansfield kind of plump. "Buxom," love that. Also, "Face Fashion," our seasonal color stories.

2:00 pm

More coffee enters my bloodstream and I call my husband to see what creation he is concocting for dinner. Apply our 100 percent Natural Lipcolor in a different shade than I applied in the am. If I could change my outfit midday, I would, but who has the time?

2:30 pm

Spend some afternoon time with the quality assurance team. Are the labels straight?

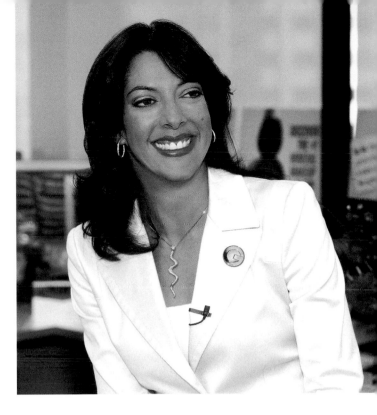

4:00 pm

Make some calls—customers, boutique managers—and check to see if the new employee luncheon is scheduled.

5:00 pm

Gather some reports and résumés to take home. (I never actually look at them, although I always think I will.)

5:45 pm

Make some phone calls on the way home—the view is tremendous—so I hang up to take it in. Get home and feel the love from all my boys—husband, son, and puppy.

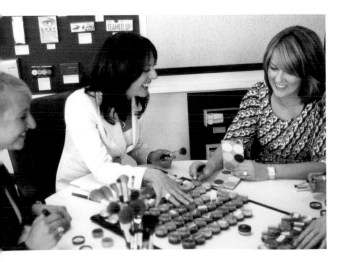

MEET JERROD BLANDINO

Get inside the ever-so-fabulous head of Too Faced creator Jerrod Blandino.

I am a self-proclaimed "culture vulture." I want to experience it all: see it, touch it, taste it, make love to it, all as fast as I can. I find inspiration in so many places. I never know when it will hit me, but when it does, I get totally obsessed.

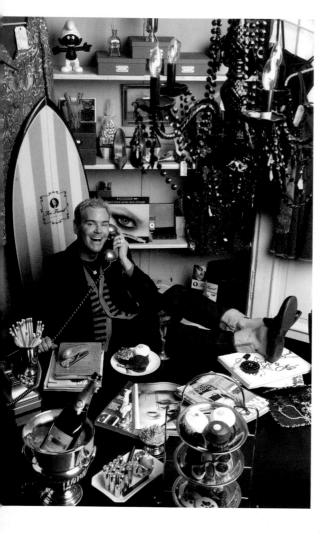

a little his-story

I grew up in the glitz and glam of the '80s, watching TV, listening to my coveted remix tape collection encompassing such lyrical gangsters as Madonna, Duran Duran, Yaz, and the Pet Shop Boys for endless inspiration. Rubber bracelets up to my elbows and Aqua Net cementing my freshly Sun-In'ed bangs into a waterfall-esque living sculpture. Those were the years when more was better. When in doubt, add something else . . . ya know?

viva la joan collins!

Alas, things couldn't stay suspended in time like an air bubble in a green gel-filled bottle of extra-strength Dippity-Do. No, I had to move forward into the bleak and cold future that was to be called "grunge." Those years of total rebellion against all that was fabulous, glamorous, or freshly washed were full of despair for me. Could it all really be over? Not while I had breath in my lungs and a bottle of Calvin Klein's Obsession for Men in my grasp!

I vowed to restore the sparkle, glitter, and gloss of my youth back to the world! So in 1998, after six years of working behind the Estée Lauder counter at Saks, I started Too Faced with my best friend, Jeremy Johnson. But enough about my past—let's get into the present. (Did someone say present? For me? Oh, you shouldn't have! Is it a diamond?)

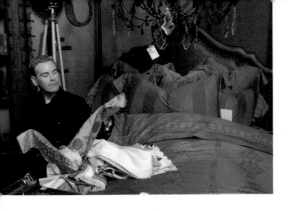

shopping for inspiration

People think creativity can be turned on and off like a switch, but it doesn't work that way. In order to get my creative juices flowing, I like to submerge myself in fashion, interior design, art, jewelry, or anything else that makes me feel connected to my creative inner eye, as well as to my customers' desires. They depend on me to tell them what's fab, what's hot, what's not, and what they'll be doing tomorrow. I have been collecting vintage Hollywood wardrobe pieces from some of my favorite films for years. Not only do the clothes inspire me, but the actresses who created such iconic characters seem to fill these garments with an indescribable energy. I am inspired by unique beauty wherever it might be found. It may be a bouquet of hot-pink tree peonies surrounded by fresh Irish shamrocks, an intricate Parisian cupcake, or a rusty gate found in an English garden that ignites that creative spark in me . . . and suddenly a lip gloss collection or new eye shadow category will develop.

baby, you're a star!

Whether I'm working with a celebrity, sorority sister, or soccer mom, I want to sprinkle a little bit of glamour into her everyday life. After all, every little girl dreams of growing up to be fabulous, doesn't she? Some may say I go a bit overboard, but I say that perhaps others hold back a bit too much. It's that simple and that complicated, but it's all TOO FACED!

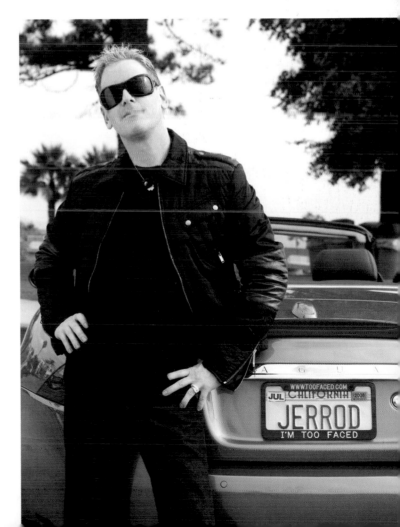

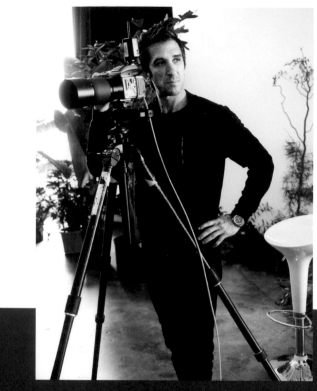

From Smashbox Cofounder and Fashion Photographer Davis Factor:
Tips on How to Take a Great Photo Every Time

- I always recommend doing your makeup in light you know you'll be going into. For instance, if you are going to a daytime BBQ, make sure you do your makeup in natural sunlight.
- Know your best features and define them for a stronger look.
- Be aware of where the light is coming from because it will mold your face. If you're looking down and the light is coming from above, then you will have dark circles. Try to move your face to where the light is flattering.
- Great posture is key!
- Always wear high heels in photo shoots, because it gives you a longer, leaner look.
- Start your makeup routine with one of the Smashbox Photo Finish Foundation Primers (I prefer the one with Dermaxyl). They smooth and balance the skin, making every photo you're in look as though it was retouched.

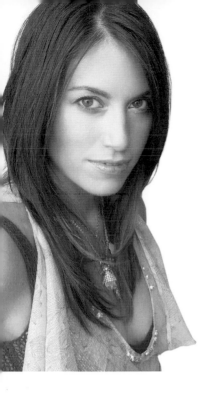

BEAUTY DIARY: WENDE ZOMNIR

At home on the beach with Urban Decay founding partner and creative director Wende Zomnir.

beauty and the beach

As the mistress of edgy, urban beauty, it may seem strange that I live at the beach—especially Newport Beach, the glitzy city featured in the TV show *The OC* . . . the place where Mercedes-Benz is as ubiquitous as Chevrolet (for the record, I drive a Lexus hybrid). But I like to call my little strip of Newport the "Newport Beach ghetto." It's a crazy mix of surfers, beach bums, homeowners, and renters. Whenever I need new ideas, I hit the boardwalk and get inspired by the craziness. And I just built a loft-inspired urban oasis right in the middle of the mayhem. A mixture of glass, steel, and concrete, it's at once a beach house and a downtown townhouse. It's a place where my edgy urban aesthetic can coexist with a beach lifestyle.

in living color

I love bold color! In my house, my clothes, and especially my makeup, of course! I have a weird orange chair and sofa that I love. I think more women should try wearing color on their eyes. It can be a soft color, but powerful at the same time—I like a muted green (Urban Decay Urb Eye shadow) or a shimmery lilac (Urban Decay Grifter Eyeshadow) to bring out the green in my hazel eyes. I get so many compliments when I bust out shades that are just a little bit dangerous for day.

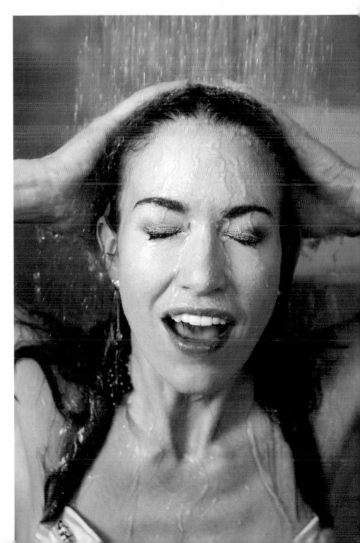

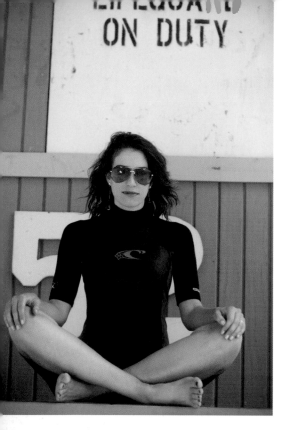

practice safe sun

Here's the best part about Newport Beach—the beach! You can surf right out my front door. And even if you don't surf, you can still have fun on the sand. I hit the beach almost daily, year round. But I never skimp on the sunscreen. I wear it in August, and I still slather it on in February. Leading an active outdoor life is so great for the body and mind, but it wreaks havoc on your skin. I put an extra dose on the tops of my hands, too. When I run on the boardwalk with my little guy in the running stroller, I try to grip the bar from the underside to keep my hands out of the sun. And I always apply an SPF 30 or more to my face, then dust it with my Urban Decay Surreal Skin Mineral Makeup. It contains titanium dioxide, so it acts as a physical block to the sun's damaging rays.

just add water

I love my outdoor shower. It's perfect for warming up after a winter's surf or rinsing off the kids coated in sand. Or just for a nice shower outside. And thanks to the power of Urban Decay Eye Shadow Primer Potion and Urban Decay Galoshes for Lashes, my eye makeup doesn't go anywhere.

boy crazy

My two amazing little boys, Crash and Cruz, are the best. Being beauty and makeup obsessed, I thought I needed a little girl to share my passion with. But my boys love mommy's purple eye shadow—they practice their painting skills with a lip brush and they create experiments with all of the pigments they find in my office. Most important, they make me feel beautiful.

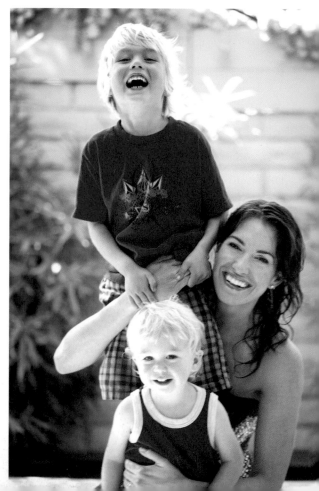

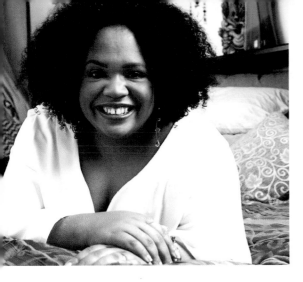

MEET LISA PRICE

Lisa Price, founder of Carol's Daughter, invites us into her Brooklyn kitchen, the birthplace of many of her beloved scrumptious body and skin care products.

If I can, I will test ideas for products out in my kitchen. The most common ingredients you'll find in my pantry are yellow beeswax and vegetable wax, cocoa butter, olive oil, toasted palm kernel oil, essential oils, and dried roses.

flower power

Whenever I get flowers—if my husband buys them for me, or if I buy them for myself—I always dry them and then I save them for potpourri or to use as decoration for when I'm putting a gift together. The proper way to dry flowers is upside down; just tie a rubber band around the stems and hang them up. The trick is to start the drying process before the head of the fresh flower starts to droop.

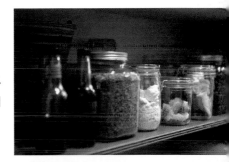

making scents

Aromatherapy is very beneficial and very powerful. My favorite oils and scents are rose, vanilla, sandalwood, patchouli, peppermint, and lavender. Roses remind me of my grandmother because she had rosebushes in her backyard. Peppermint is very refreshing; I'll add it to anything because it cools you and it doesn't distort any other fragrance. I like to massage with a body rub that has eucalyptus and peppermint oil if I have a cold. And I have bath salts called Body Aches, which are made with lavender and peppermint. When I'm sick, if I have the energy I soak in a bath with the salts, but if I don't have the energy, I sprinkle it on the shower floor so the shower becomes a steam with the lavender and peppermint.

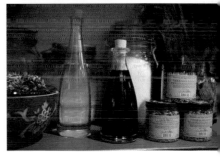

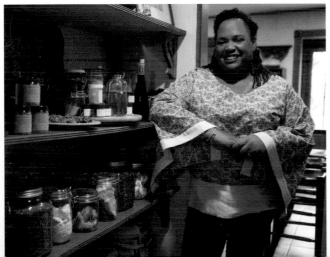

scrub at home

I make body scrubs with sea salt and fruit, but it's not something I can sell because it's perishable. I may mix sea salt with fresh lime juice, shredded pineapples, and coconut oil. You get exfoliation from the fruit and salt, and the coconut oil moisturizes.

smooth as butter

I keep chunks of shea and cocoa butter in a jar. Real cocoa butter smells like chocolate and is great for itchy or dry skin. Shea butter really works on any part of the body as a soothing and protective moisturizer. I get my shea butter imported from West Africa.

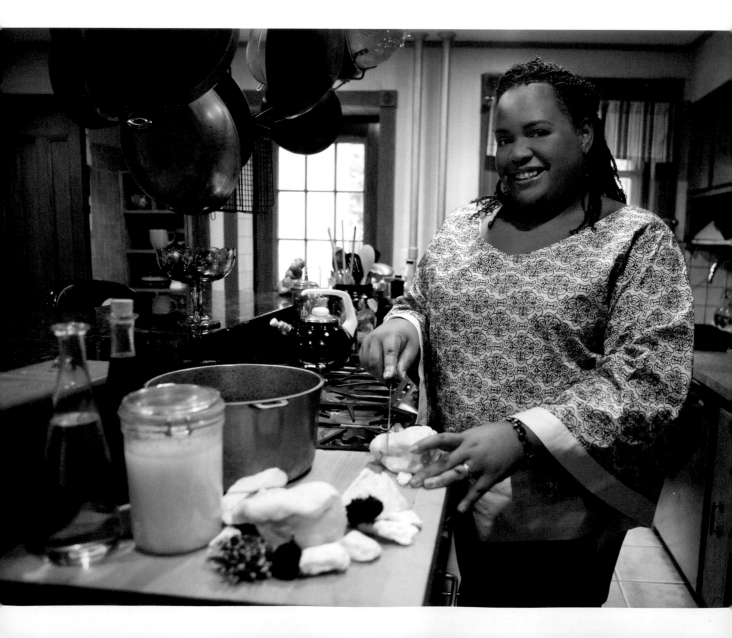

BEAUTY DIARY: MAUREEN KELLY

Spend a day in the life with Tarte founder Maureen Kelly.

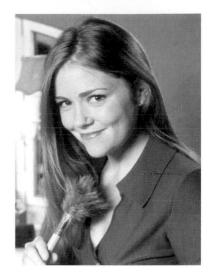

6:15 am

My son, Sully, is my alarm clock—when he wakes up, so do I! These days the circles under my eyes are getting darker and looking more puffy than usual. I've found that placing a slightly warmed tea bag (chamomile is my favorite) over my eyes for about ten minutes wakes me up.

7:30 am

Most mornings I have an egg-white omelet with spinach and cheese, multigrain toast with jam, and a glass of Sambazon's acai juice.

8:25 am

I've definitely mastered the "ten minute or less" shower—I cleanse with a mild, natural scented soap or body wash. Once out of the shower, I apply baby oil to my skin while it's still damp. It's the ultimate moisturizer. I've also started using BORBA's Fiber-Knit Diamond Shimmer Body Contour mixed with a few extra drops of vitamin E oil on my tummy to prevent stretch marks.

9:15 am

Sure, I own a cosmetics company, but I spend only five minutes getting ready in the morning. I keep my routine simple:
• Our Eraser Concealer is really my magical eraser—with a few swipes I can hide those dark circles (thanks to vitamin E and Arnica), eliminate any signs of puffy eyes, and cover redness.
• I dab Tipsy Cheek Stain to help me fake that "pregnancy glow."
• Then I layer on Tarte Lights! Camera! Lashes! 4-in-1 Mascara. My senses are a bit heightened these days so I lightly spritz a fresh-scented perfume (I'm into Frederic Malle Lys Méditerranée at the moment).

10:15 am

The first thing I do when I get into the office is light some candles. One of my absolute favorites is Calypso's Mimosa candle. It gives me a sense of calmness and helps me focus on the day's work.

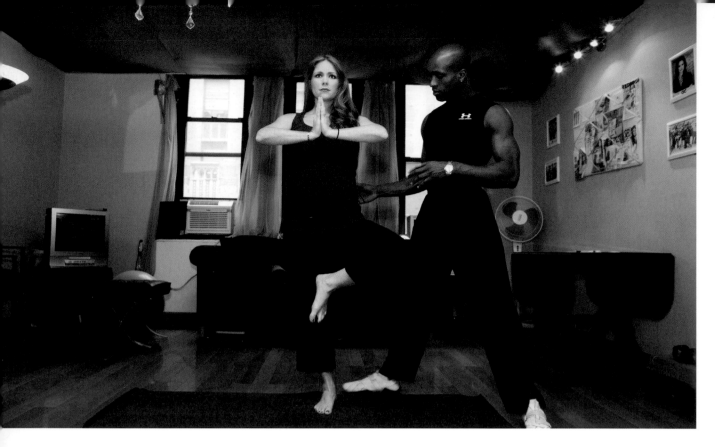

12:15

Since I'm always testing new Tarte colors and natural formulas from the labs on my hands, you'll always find me applying and reapplying L'Occitane Shea Butter hand cream. It helps prevent dry and irritated skin.

3:00 pm

We have our daily Tarte meeting—these tend to get stressful, so I keep essential oils by my desk. I mix them together and then massage my temples while we discuss everything going on.

5:30 pm

Right now, I'm all about yoga. I love the fluidity of the poses. With so much going on in my life, it really puts me at ease while also being a great workout.

6:30 pm

Before leaving the office, I spray Evian mineral water spray on my face and then use Mustela's Hydra-Stick on my lips and cheeks. I carry this all-purpose balm everywhere I go—it's great for my son, too!

7:45 pm

Once we tuck our little guy into bed, I take a warm bath (not hot) with a few drops of Aveeno's Active Naturals Stress Relief Body Wash—it contains the relaxing scents of lavender, ylang-ylang, and chamomile.

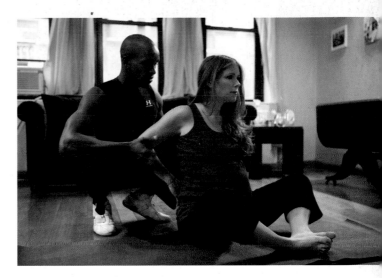

10:00 pm

To soothe my achy legs and tired feet, I massage them with my own little treat. I add a few drops of peppermint oil to my moisturizer. It has such a cooling effect and leaves a nice healthy glow. I also reapply pure cocoa butter all over my baby bump before I fall asleep.

Maureen's Tips on How to Look and Feel Gorgeous Throughout Pregnancy

- Get a bimonthly facial—it will help with breakouts and blotchy skin.
- Pamper yourself to the fullest: get regular prenatal massages.
- Manicures and pedicures are a definite must-have! Even if everything else is disheveled, that leaves me feeling polished.
- If stressed, light a candle, dab an essential oil on the temples, or take a freshly scented bath.

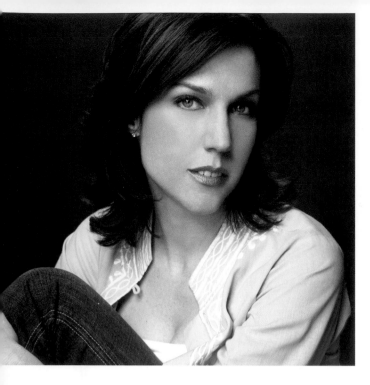

MASTER STASHES: CRISTINA BARTOLUCCI

Take a peek inside the bag of celebrity makeup artist and DuWop cofounder Cristina Bartolucci.

binaca

When you're doing makeup, it's such an intimate thing: you're touching someone, you're up in their face, and the last thing you want is bad breath!

ben nye translucent powder

This is a colorless powder in a shaker. It's very basic and it works really well. I just tap a little bit out on the table and dab the brush in and give the T-zone a quick once-over with it at the end. Because of its whiteish color, I am extra-careful about how much I use. When you're working with a colored powder, there's a tendency to use too much because it matches the skin, but true translucent powder, with a white tinge to it, is a visual reminder to go light. I try to pull out as much of the oil as possible with blotting papers first, and then as a last resort, I use powder.

duwop bronze rush

I want to give everybody a very clean, sharp jawline and I find a really natural way to contour is to dip a big, fluffy brush into the bronzer, twirl it underneath the chin, and then work it down onto the chest. It's completely undetectable, but it really makes a difference. I also find that using a bronzer around the hairline and below the cheekbone helps to sculpt the face. This bronzer doesn't get cakey and it has just the right amount of shimmer. I use the cheek stain as the base for whatever cheek I'm doing. Sometimes, when I want just a kiss of color, I'll use it alone, but when I want to do something

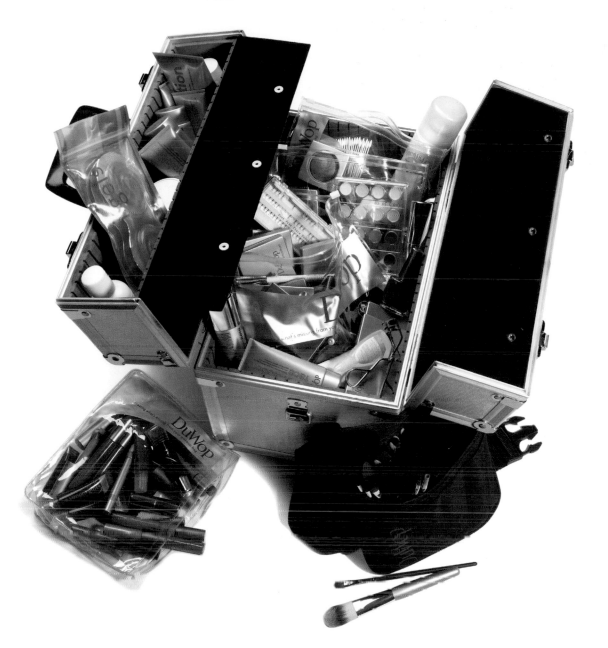

more elaborate, I'll put the stain on underneath and then I'll work a light powder blush over it, like Nars Orgasm, then DuWop Blush Booster over that. Layered cheeks are very in right now. Layering different finishes of sheer blush on the cheek gives them dimensions and really highlights the cheekbone.

laura mercier palette

This has real sentimental value to me. The palette was one of the first collections Laura Mercier put out. The colors are so beautiful in it and it was the first time I really had money to spend on really nice makeup, so this was my first splurge. Even though the mirror is cracked, I still love and use the colors. I refuse to think of the cracked mirror as bad luck!

tea tree oil

I will put a touch of tea tree oil on a blemish at the beginning of doing someone's makeup. It disinfects it and will stop it from festering underneath whatever I'm doing. It takes the wind out of blemishes.

duwop blush booster

Probably my current favorite DuWop product. It puts your cheeks into hyperdrive. Whatever blush you're wearing—whether it's cream or powder—put this over it! I like to run a blush brush over Blush Booster and then smush the brush all the way in and run it along your cheekbone. It's going to catch the light and is in keeping with the whole idea of layering your cheek. It's also really versatile in terms of the application. I like to brush it over eye makeup— it kicks it up to the next level. My favorite color is Apple, which is a pinkish nude. I like to put a tiny bit on the décolletage as well.

badger balm

I use it on lips and anywhere the skin needs some moisture. It smells really good!

shu uemura eyelash curler

This is such a cliché for makeup artists, but I couldn't live without this tool. With other lash curlers I've used, the curl goes away five minutes later, but not with this one. If you get in right at the lashline with this sucker, it will stay. I like to crimp once really hard and then I get that big, open eye, then the crimp slowly relaxes into a nice curve.

duwop brown eye kit

I created this because it's what I needed as a makeup artist. I tried to make it as user-friendly as possible. You have all of these colors and all of these possibilities. You can mix and play, but you can't go wrong. It's every form of brown eye shadow possible. You can do anything from the most sleek, subtle daytime look to a big, bold, glamorous smoky eye.

foundation brush

We created this for our artists in the field, so we don't currently sell it. I use it to put on tinted moisturizer in five minutes. It's soft, it feels good, and I can use it on the body.

duwop revolotion

This gives a little more coverage than your average tinted moisturizer, and it has a satin matte rather than dewy finish. If I can get away with it, I'll just use this on the complexion and nothing else.

visine

This is a staple! Sometimes when you're working on a smoky eye, you can unintentionally irritate someone's eyes. You don't want to get done with a beautiful look and then have it ruined with bloodshot eyes.

nars lip palette in hot sauce

By mixing the colors in this palette, I can pretty much create any deeper shade of lipstick I need. I like the texture of it and the colors look good on almost anyone.

lip venom

Sometimes on shoots, I won't want the model or actress to be distracted by the feeling of Lip Venom, so I'll just use it as a plumper and then wipe it off and do her lips. But in real life, it's fantastic, because you kind of want that feeling where you're pouty and aware of your lips.

duwop real lipstick in josephine

This is named after Josephine Baker, who is a strong female icon. I love this color because it's a little bit neutral and it works on all skin tones. It will turn a little bit of a berry on a light-skin girl and it will read as a pale neutral on a darker skin tone.

sponge

I never use sponges to wipe the face, but sometimes I'll use them to pat something in or to clean up under the eyes.

candle

A little signature I like to have at my makeup station. It creates a little bit of atmosphere. Models and actresses get so scrutinized in front of the camera, so I like to create a calming, peaceful haven for them.

shiseido creamy blush in rambler rose

This color has just enough shimmer in it and it's a pretty raspberry color. I'm a big Shiseido fan.

duwop duet gloss and highlighter

A nice way to add life to the face and to know that your gloss is going to go really well with your highlighter.

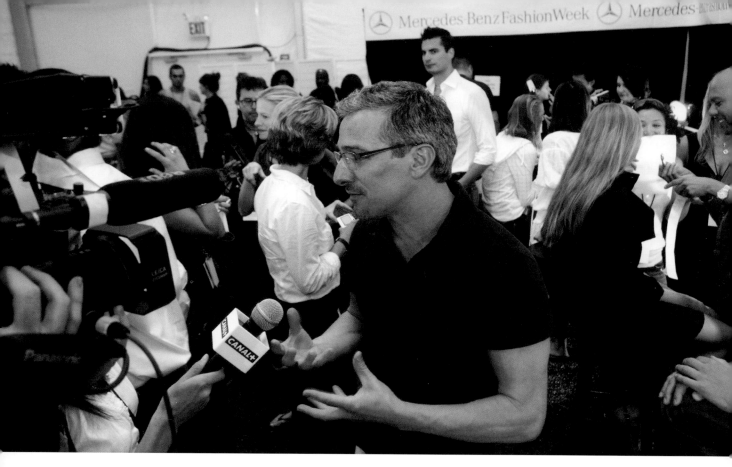

BEAUTY DIARY: VINCENT LONGO

Experience the madness, mayhem, and molto *makeup backstage during New York Fashion Week with Vincent Longo.*

I've been doing makeup at fashion shows since 1982 in Milan. I was a twenty-year-old junior artist running around backstage at Gianfranco Ferré, Versace, Armani, and Dolce & Gabbana. The shows are part of my DNA at this point! Fashion shows are full of excitement—it's where real moments of creativity occur. Nowadays, I'm very selective with the designers I choose to work with. I prefer to work with younger designers, because they give more space to creativity and it helps me keep my finger on the pulse. This season I chose to work with designer Erin Fetherston, a real up-and-coming force in the fashion industry.

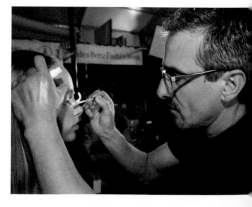

a couple days before the show

I first meet with Erin at her studio on 42nd Street. Clothes are everywhere and there's a lot of creative momentum happening. She walks me through the collection and starts talking about her inspiration. The idea is to get an overall creative feel on where the designer is coming from. I try to find a parallel with my makeup collection that I'm working on for that same period. The goal is to try to match those creative juices and bring them together in a collectiveness that translates into something interesting. There's a lot of white in her collection and she tells me she was thinking about a beauty that was unexpected and a little whimsical. All of a sudden it all came together. I had white mascara and white liner coming out for spring/summer and it married perfectly with her theme.

show day

8 am
I wake up after dreaming about white mascara last night! This isn't unusual—I dream about products a lot. Recently I had a dream where I was creating colors in a lab.

8:45 am
Over my breakfast, I start getting really excited, because it's not that common to be able to do a fashion show in New York that's innovative, forward-thinking, and truly on the pulse with what's happening in beauty.

9:45 am
There's a traffic jam, plus a cab strike. I'm on my Vespa with my makeup kit sitting between my legs and I can't even get through 23rd Street!

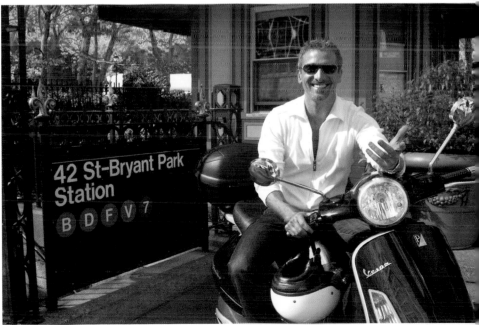

10:30 am

I arrive twenty minutes after call time. Which is fine, because we made the call time a little earlier anyway. I'm racing into Bryant Park. I'm on the cell phone with my assistant, and she comes to meet me outside the tents and races me inside. I forgot the invitation (with the location entrance details) at home.

10:45 am

I check out the lay of the land and check in on my assistants to see what they're doing. I set up my station. I start finding out if everything's OK with hair, because our teams work in tandem. The first thing I need to do is re-create the look on a model that I created for Erin in her showroom. That way, she can reconfirm that what I'm about to do with the whole team is exactly what she's looking for. I discover that the first model sitting in my chair is Marie—I had used her in my own photo shoot the previous year!

11:15 am

Uh oh! There's a problem with our key product—the white mascara. The bags they were traveling in from my office to Bryant Park broke on the way and all the contents (tissues, the mascara, makeup remover) went scattering all over Sixth Avenue. My team has to go back to my offices and repack the bags with new

products. I'm already delayed because I was late—now there's this! I start to panic. If you get too far behind once you're backstage, it's treacherous, because catching up is a nightmare. I'm starting to lose it . . .

11:25 am

Phew! My team shows up with the mascara. We're able to move forward. Erin sees the look and loves it straightaway. We start moving with the hair and makeup team exchanging the models.

noon

The camera crews start descending. I love doing interviews, but I'm sweating them a bit because there have been a few hiccups. I see some of the makeup artists have gone a little too heavy on the brows, and now I need to go soften them up. The first looks are about to happen and I don't want Erin to see that a few girls look off. I send my nephew, who's my right hand, to do a round with all the girls. My eye is concentrated on what's happening with the models, but I'm getting a lot of journalists coming at me for interviews right at the same moment. I want to say hold up, but I can't when there's a whole camera crew. They need access now. This is when I start juggling.

12:45 pm

Finally, the makeup is perfect. It's really exciting to see the culmination of getting all these girls ready. I love seeing twenty beautiful women all lined up with the same look, the same hair, flowing with the collection—it's harmonized in the most beautiful way. It's such an exhilarating moment. There's so much electricity in the air right before the first look goes out onto the runway.

1:00 pm: show starts

I stand right beside Erin next to the exit of the runway with the hairstylist. The designer is the one who touches the models last before she goes out and the hairstylist and makeup artist are right there with her. I need to make sure that every girl who goes out is matte and well-powdered and that everything about her beauty is spot-on. If she needs retouching with lip gloss, or if her body needs moisturizing, I have two other assistants standing by with me to do the job.

1:15 pm: show ends

Once the finale happens, I make sure Erin is powdered and lip glossed so she can take her bow. I congratulate Erin on a great collection. Then I go back and congratulate and thank the production team and my team for doing a great job. I immediately start feeling the pressure releasing and the tension coming down. I start breathing again. I think to myself it's over . . . until next season.

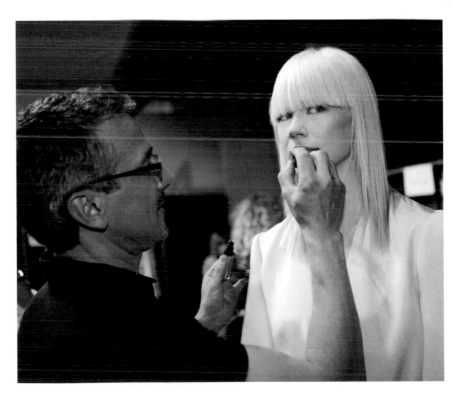

MASTER STASHES: OSCAR BLANDI

Celebrity hairstylist and owner of one of New York's hottest salons Oscar Blandi gives us a look inside his kit.

velcro rollers

I love Velcro rollers, because they have more flexibility and grab on to the hair much better than other rollers. You don't need clips to secure these, so there's no line of demarcation. But you always have to be careful when removing them. I always like to hold on to the section of hair when you're removing the roller because it's still grabbing the hair and it can create frizz.

round brush

This is one of the easiest tools for everybody to use. I like to use bristles that are a mix between natural boar and plastic, because the plastic will hold the hair and the boar will smooth down the hair shaft and maximize the shine.

scissors

I usually bring five or six pairs of scissors with me to jobs. These are my thinning shears. The teeth are wider than normal to create chunky pieces. They help give a shaggy, wispy, sexy, piecey look to the hair.

twin turbo blow dryer

I've been using this blow dryer for many years. For me, I need a hair dryer to give me heat, speed, and the right shape. I always make sure to protect the hair with Jasmine Oil Serum in conjunction with other products to create a barrier on the hair. To give the hair shape, take a section, roll it underneath with a round brush, keep the dryer on the section, do the rolling motion several times, and leave the brush rolled in there for a few moments. This is when actual shape will happen. The hair gets hot during the blow-drying process, so you really have to let it cool off in a specific shape to give it a style.

oscar blandi riccia curling serum

This is one of my favorite products—I use it on myself all the time! It was created because I was looking at women with curly hair and their hair always looks better when it's wet. When it starts to dry, the hair gets fuzzy, frizzy, and big. What Riccia does is gives the curl that wet look without being crunchy. It's not only containing the curl, but it's conditioning it as well.

oscar blandi no gravity volumizing spray

I worked really hard and long to make this product. In the early '90s, I would do photo shoots for *Cosmopolitan* that would require really big hair. I would use protein, which strengthened the hair, but it always made it so sticky. I wanted something to make hair really sexy and voluminous, but would also allow a brush to glide through it. You can use this on wet hair and dry hair.

oscar blandi pronto dry shampoo spray

This product helps me on photo shoots when there's not always time to wash someone's hair. It removes all the impurities and reveals a fresh layer of hair. This is a temporary wash, but it really cleans and softens the hair. Like a mint to freshen your breath, it refreshes your scalp and prolongs washing for another day or two.

oscar blandi tempo hair treatment trio

This is a trio of my best treatment products. I created this kit as a tool for people to understand what the hair needs to be healthy. It contains:

Jasmine Smoothing Hair Treatment

This is a frizz-fighter that will even help fight frizz in humidity. It's an intense conditioning agent that really repairs the hair. The more you do it, the more beneficial it will be.

Exfoliating Treatment

You should exfoliate your hair once a week, the same way you exfoliate your skin. Just like with skin, there's product buildup that needs to be removed. All your other hair products will work better afterward, and your hair will become more radiant and will have more life. Not only will this give you a nice gentle cleansing, but your hair will be infused with vitamins. It will also help with any damage the hair already has. If you use this once a week, you'll see results within a month. Improving the hair takes time.

Fango

This is really, really strong stuff. It's made for all hair types, but specifically for seriously damaged, overprocessed hair. Fango goes right into the hair shaft and builds a barrier, so it will protect your hair from any impurities trying to get in. This treatment is great for someone who is this close to cutting their hair off and wants to bring back the healthy hair they had once upon a time.

MEET OLE HENRIKSEN

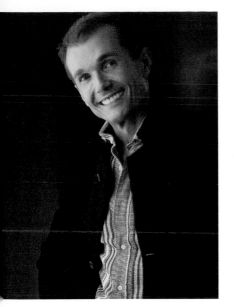

Danish skin care guru Ole Henriksen is the picture of health, vitality, and glowing skin. His secret is to practice old-time Scandinavian rituals and a less-is-more approach to life.

I find incorporating certain aspects of my Scandinavian heritage into my everyday life helps me to fight stress and remain positive and energetic. Whether it's the way I prepare my meals (simple and healthy) or the way I pack my suitcase (by choosing a theme of two colors, so I'm never left confused), it's all about sticking to the basics and doing them faithfully. Following a less-is-more approach to life keeps me happy, healthy, and focused on the moment. Here are my secrets.

cold water therapy

In Scandinavia, it's amazing how many people—young and old—break the ice during the winter and go swimming. It must be the Viking part of our blood. Over the years, I've learned the power of cold water—it truly awakens and revives the skin. My little trick is to pour a tray of ice cubes into a sink full of cold water, dip a terry facecloth into it, and then lay it across the face for a few moments. This is a great way to oxygenate and lift the skin—it's like a mini face-lift.

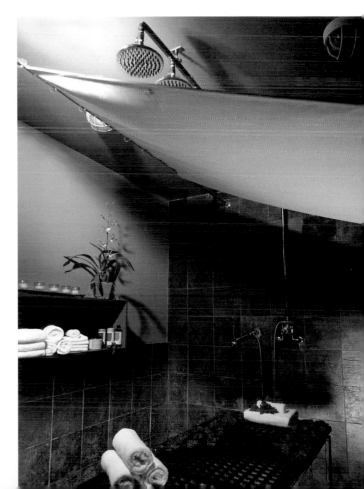

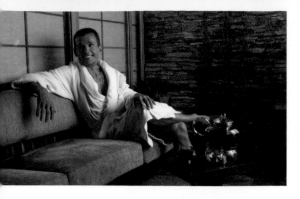

tea time

I like to turn ordinary moments into something special. Such is the case with my morning tea, which I make into a beautiful ritual with a nice presentation of flowers, china I love, and a nutritious homemade breakfast. It really sets the tone for the day.

office space

Creating a peaceful environment at work is so important. I always like to have something green on my desk. Bamboo is a wonderful choice, because it's beautiful, sculptural, and grows in any kind of light, or lack thereof.

quiet, please

We don't always need to have an iPod stuck in our ears. As human beings, we have a need for peace and quiet. So much creativity flows and so many answers come to us in those moments of quiet.

get physical

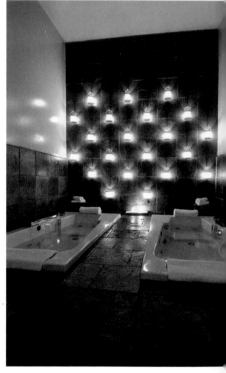

Physical activity was a big part of my entire upbringing. The Danish use bicycles as their main mode of transportation. As an adult, I've learned exercise provides new energy and is key in fighting stress, the greatest enemy of our health and our looks. Depending on my schedule I will either do a twenty-minute or forty-five-minute workout, but I do it faithfully. My routines involve a lot of stretching, and working against my own body weight (push-ups and sit-ups), so I'm not dependent on fancy equipment, and I put on my favorite music and dance for my cardio. People think you need a trainer or a gym membership, but you don't! I live in the Hollywood Hills and I see the major movie stars out running with their dogs—so even the rich and famous stay in shape without expert help.

saltwater

Sea salt is a very simple cure for treating tired and fatigued muscles. I like to take candlelit baths and really create my own ambience in my bathroom. Candles are a big part of the Scandinavian culture, because it's so dark there. You really don't need to go to a spa to pamper yourself—you can do it at home. Here's how: Take a pint of Epsom salts, blend into warm water, add a half ounce of eucalyptus essential oil, and three ounces of almond oil. Stir together. The eucalyptus aroma has uplifting benefits and the fat of the almond oil will add that protective mantle, so when you step out of the bath, you will have really soft skin. Roll a hand towel under your neck. Lay back and soak.

food for life

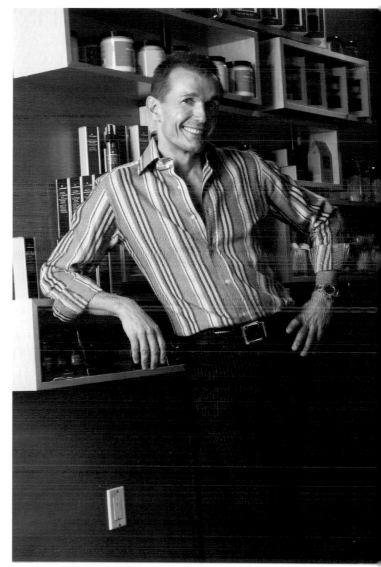

Nutrition is something my mom put a lot of emphasis on when I was growing up. Sweets were a special treat—given to us only once a week. Eating healthy, delicious foods is something I do every single day, even when I travel! When it's a morning flight, I bring a Tupperware container with oatmeal, flaxseed, and raw almonds to the airport, and add hot milk or water from Starbucks. Then, to take on the flight, I'll make a multigrain sandwich with almond butter and mashed bananas, and a side of avocado, sprouts, and a little cheese. Healthy fats are vital for brain function, eyesight, and for the quality of your hair and skin. They also provide amazing energy, because fat is burned slowly.

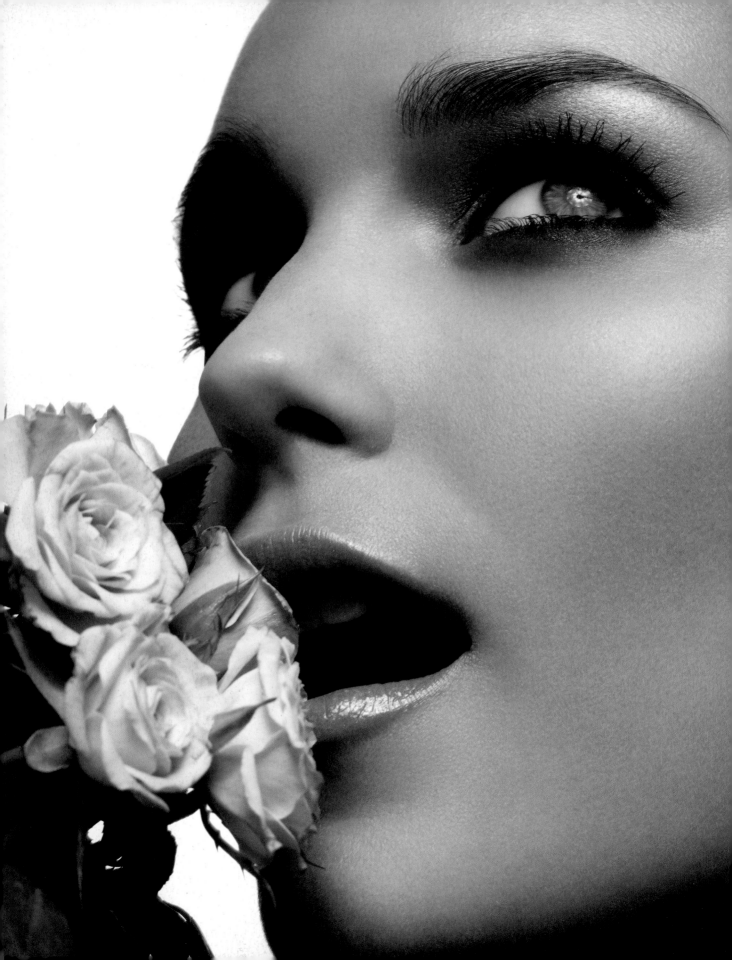

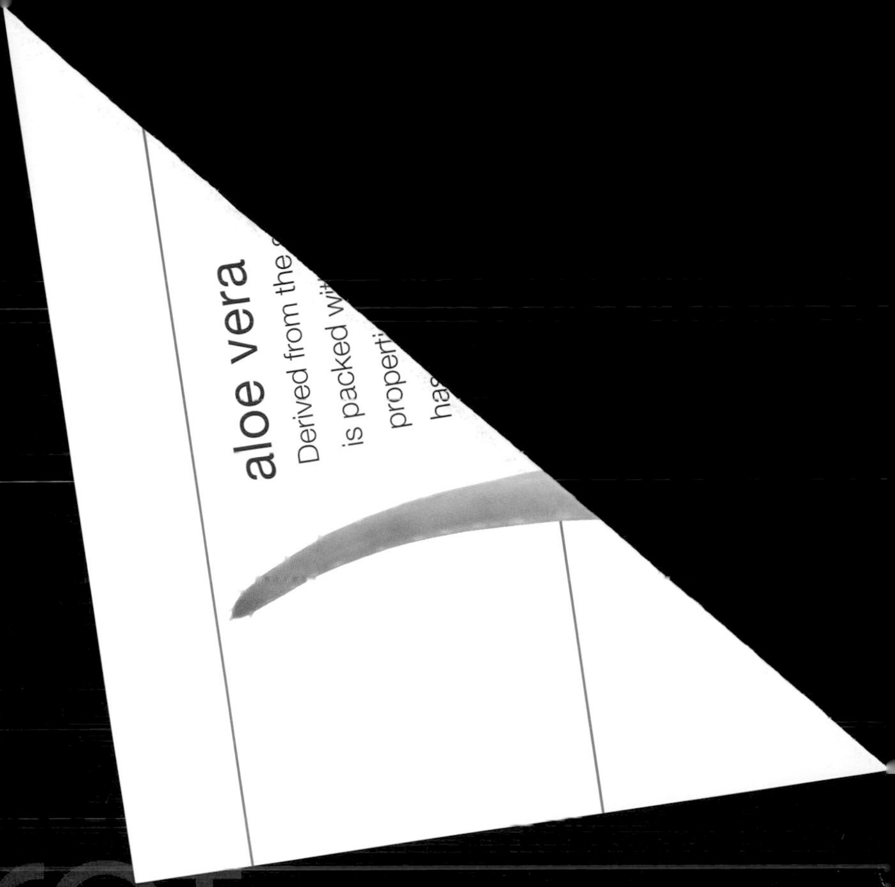

aloe vera

Derived from the [...]
is packed wi[...]
properti[...]
ha[...]

secret
ingredients

Spread your smarts after discovering the definitions of those highfalutin', hard-to-pronounce names found in many cosmetics.

acai

What's been a staple in the diets of Brazilian natives for years is a hot new skin-saving ingredient. Acai (pronounced *ah-sigh-ee*) is a powerful antioxidant that's being boldly touted as one of the most nutritious fruits around. Harvested from the Amazon, this tiny berry boasts a résumé of seriously impressive powers. The most intriguing to the beauty world is its ability to smooth and soften skin while helping to eliminate toxins.

short-stemmed aloe plant indigenous to Africa, aloe vera
with hydrating, healing, anti-inflammatory, and antimicrobial
properties. Because of its immediate refreshing and relaxing effect, aloe vera
has been used to treat burns for hundreds of years and is still used today in
post-sun care.

alpha hydroxy acid (aha)

AHA is the family name for a variety of acids: citric acid, glycolic acid,
lactic acid, malic acid, and tartaric acid. Centuries ago, women seeking
younger-looking skin would apply acidic ingredients, such as old wine,
sour milk, or lemon juice to their faces. Legend has it that Cleopatra
bathed in sour milk (lactic acid) to improve her complexion. Nowadays,
these naturally occurring acids, called alpha hydroxy acids, are
sophistically formulated and added to numerous skin-care
products. Lactic and glycolic acid are the most common
and effective forms used in anti-aging and anti-acne
products, as they remove the flaky, "dead" layer
of skin from the epidermis (the skin's outermost
layer) to improve the skin's texture and color and
speed up cell renewal.

alpha lipoic acid (ala)

ALA's nickname, the "universal antioxidant," comes from the fact that it dissolves in both
water and fat. Its unique structure makes it supereasy to enter cell membranes, fight free
radicals, and energize the cells, hence the reason it's found in many anti-aging creams. ALA
is an effective anti-inflammatory that works to improve microcirculation and is currently being
studied as a treatment for diabetes.

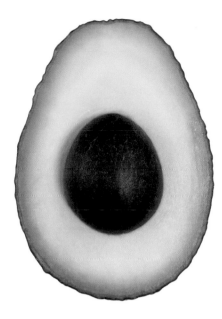

avocado

An essential fatty acid that treats the skin from the inside and out, avocado is used in many natural and organic skin-care products because its antibacterial properties work well as a preservative. Avocado is also highly emollient, so it provides slip and creaminess to products, making them soothing on the skin. These pulpy green fruits are true beauty foods—they're packed with antioxidants and healthy fats, which keep the skin glowing and youthful.

amino acids

Found in all forms of life, amino acids are the body's building blocks. In terms of beauty, amino acids enhance water retention in the skin and keep products moist, preventing them from drying out. Many amino acids come from animal collagen, but new vegetable alternatives are making their way into the market.

beta hydroxy acid (bha)

Commonly referred to as salicylic acid, BHA helps shed the skin's cells and refine the texture. BHA is an amazing ingredient for acne-prone skin, as it's extremely effective in reducing clogged pores and breakouts through exfoliation.

chamomile

Chamomile, a flowering herb derived from an aromatic white or yellow flower, is the ultimate soother. Used in teas and cosmetics for its anti-inflammatory, antiseptic, and skin-softening properties, chamomile helps neutralize any skin irritants. It's also hypoallergenic and noncomedogenic, so sensitive skin types can feel safe using it in their skin care.

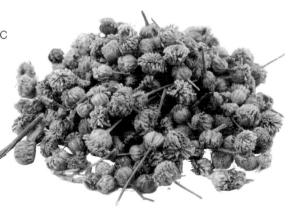

cocoa butter

A cream-colored, fatty substance derived from the roasted seeds of the cacao plant. Cocoa butter melts below body temperature, making it an excellent lubricant for lip balms and body creams.

co-enzyme q10 (coq10)

This naturally occurring antioxidant is found in all human cells as well as in meats; fish; and soybean, sesame, and canola oils. In addition to combating free radical damage to the skin, it works to "jump start" cell metabolism by increasing oxygenation and energy production in the cells. As we age, levels of CoQ10 in the skin diminish, resulting in lesser ability to produce collagen and elastin and making our skin more prone to free radical damage. So CoQ10 in skin care works as a great anti-aging treatment.

cornstarch

Finely ground corn kernels used in powders and powder foundations to absorb moisture and oil and mattify the skin.

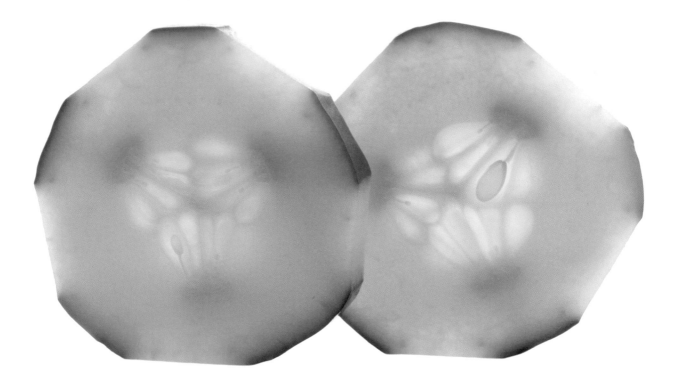

cucumber extract

A natural humectant, cucumber extract has loads of benefits. From soothing and softening the skin to providing instant anti-inflammatory refreshment, cucumber extract is a dream ingredient. Other tricks it can do are tighten stressed-out skin and depuff tired eyes.

dihydroxyacetone (dha)

Self-tanners wouldn't exist without DHA, as it's the ingredient that turns the skin a golden brown sans the sun. DHA is a color additive that reacts with the amino acids on the skin and colors the skin a deeper shade mimicking a suntan.

evening primrose oil

Named evening primrose because its light yellow flowers open at dusk, evening primrose oil is a source of gamma-linoleic acid, an essential fatty acid. The body converts evening primrose oil into a hormone-like substance, which regulates a number of bodily functions. It has an anti-inflammatory effect that protects against cardiovascular disease and arthritis. It's also used in the treatment of eczema, acne, dermatitis, asthma, and allergies. Evening primrose oil can also alleviate the symptoms of PMS and is thought to reduce cholesterol and high blood pressure.

glycerin

A skin conditioning agent and softener often found in facial cleansing products, cuticle oils, face creams, and lotions, glycerin is a syrupy liquid formed by the decomposition of oil, fats, and molasses. Glycerin is a natural humectant that keeps products moist, makes them spread more easily, and prevents evaporation of water from the skin. Glycerin is especially effective on chapped skin.

goji berry

These Tibetan berries are loaded with essential fatty acids, antioxidants, minerals, more beta-carotene, and 500 times more vitamin C than oranges. Goji berries have long been used in traditional Chinese medicine to give the immune system a boost and improve circulation. When used in topical skin care, gojis help to treat redness, sensitivity, and inflammation.

grapeseed oil

An excellent antioxidant that helps to prevent the breakdown of collagen and elastin fibers. The high linoleic acid content helps promote skin smoothness, which is why it's often found in lip balm, hand creams, and other hydrating products.

green tea

One of the best antioxidants around, green tea is responsible for warding off many diseases in the body—even cancer. Due to its anti-inflammatory, antioxidant properties, green tea extract is found in many anti-aging treatments. This wonder tea can also extend the SPF ability in skin-care products.

jojoba oil

Jojoba oil is derived from the seed of the jojoba plant, a shrub found in desert regions. Its makeup is very close to the skin's natural oils, which makes it noncomedogenic and a fantastic skin lubricant. Jojoba oil also provides great spreadability to cream cosmetics.

kaolin

This white soft powder (also called China cla typically found in face powder, powder blush baby powder, and some foundations. It absorbs water and oil and adheres well to the skin's surface.

lavender oil

An all-around amazing oil, lavender has antibacterial, antiseptic, astringent, healing, and purifying qualities. It's been proven to rel anxiety, stress, and can even help induce sle When used in skin care, lavender oil can red redness and blotchiness, while calming and overactive and acne skins. It also helps to pr stretch marks.

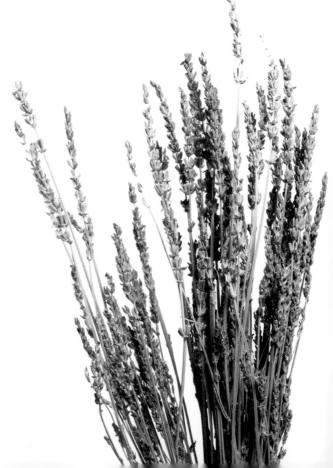

meadowfoam

The oil from the meadowfoam plant has a unique fatty acid composition that helps the skin retain its natural moisture level. It's used in everything from mascara and eye shadow to suntan lotion and shampoo for its moisturizing capabilities.

mica

Derived from pearls, fish scales or rocks, mica is what gives shimmer and luminosity to many makeup products.

neuropeptides

Though they sound like science geeks, neuropeptides are actually the body's social butterflies. A huge player in our internal communication network, neuropeptides act as chemical messengers between the brain and the body. When we're young, our skin is full of anti-inflammatory neuropeptides, which signal the brain to keep cell turnover speedy, but as we age, these neuropeptides diminish.

parsol 1789

Also known as avobenzone, Parsol 1789 the damaging effects of both UVA and U which cause wrinkles and hyperpigment

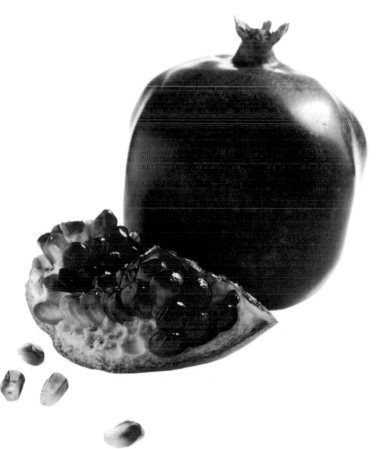

peppermint

An anti-irritant, antibacterial herb that hel redness and skin irritation from acne. Its and refreshing properties help to relieve redness and irritation by constricting capillaries, so it's great for ruddy skin tones.

pomegranate

Just like green tea and red wine, pomegranates contain extremely high levels of polyphenols: powerful antioxidants that help stabilize free radicals, which cause premature aging. In fact, pomegranates are one of mankind's oldest medications. The Greek physician Hippocrates used the fruit to soothe eye irritations and aid digestion. Now new research has shown that pomegranates may be one of the most potent wrinkle-fighters.

pumice

Best known for sloughing off rough skin, pumice is a highly porous volcanic rock. Pumice powder is used in acne products as a strong exfoliant.

rose water

Rose water is loved for its soothing, nourishing, and rejuvenating properties. It has a calming effect on skin ailments, such as eczema and psoriasis, and is both antiseptic and anti-inflammatory.

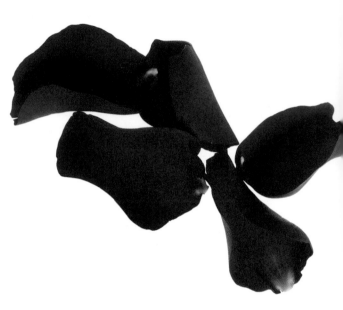

rosemary

Its astringent, toning, antiseptic, and stimulating properties make it beneficial in cellulite treatments. It increases circulation and is extremely helpful for treating oily skin.

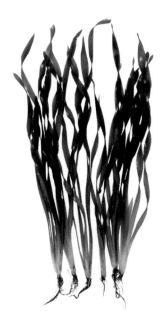

salicylic acid

A natural ingredient found in some plants, such as wintergreen leaves and sweet birch, this BHA improves the appearance and condition of the skin by removing the dead cells from the epidermis, allowing new cells to rise to the surface. Salicylic acid is highly effective in acne-fighting products.

seaweed

This marine plant has garnered many fans for its healing, moisturizing, and protective properties. Seaweed is anti-inflammatory due to its high sulfur and amino acid content. Great for treating aging and dry skin, seaweed also improves blood circulation, which is why it's found in many anti-cellulite treatments.

shea butter

Known as a natural moisturizer, shea butter is a natural lipid that comes from the fruit of the karite tree. It's a vitamin-rich, antioxidant best known for keeping skin baby soft, healing burns or wounds, and promoting cell regeneration. As skin friendly as ingredients come, shea butter penetrates deeply and is easily absorbed (so it doesn't clog pores), aids in sun protection, helps prevent premature aging, and increases skin's moisture to a butter-soft level.

silica

A naturally occurring white powder found in 12 percent of all rocks, silica is mainly found in many sunscreens and toiletries.

soy

Extracted from soybeans and soy milk, this high-protein ingredient has recently become a favorite for anti-aging products. These proteins are known for containing high levels of antioxidants.

sulfur

A natural, nonmetallic element found in meat, fish, poultry, eggs, milk, legumes, onions, brussels sprouts, and cabbage, sulfur is necessary for the formation of collagen and binds protein molecules in hair, fingernails and toenails, and skin. Sulfur is often used as a topical antiseptic acne treatment because it is effective in drying excess sebum.

sweet almond oil

Formulated from sweet almonds that have been cleaned, crushed, and cold-pressed. It's an emollient used in creams, lotions, and bath oils to give a slippery-smooth, luxurious feeling.

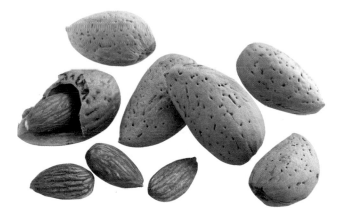

talc

This finely ground, naturally occurring mineral (magnesium silicate) is used in many loose powders to help absorb oil and set makeup.

tea tree oil

This natural and highly antiseptic preservative derived from the Australian tea tree plant has been used for many centuries to treat cuts and wounds. Today it's still widely used in treating a host of skin infections, such as eczema, dermatitis, and psoriasis.

titanium dioxide

A nonchemical UVA and UVB ray blocker, titanium dioxide is a powerful SPF contributor that stays on the skin's surface and scatters UV light. When the particles are large, it can leave a whitish hue on the skin; when particles are more elegant, barely a trace of color can be seen.

vitamin a (beta carotene, retinol)

This fat-soluble unsaturated alcohol, found in green and yellow vegetables, egg yolks, butter, and fish-liver oils, is an important vitamin required for healthy skin, both internally and externally. Vitamin A is a powerful antioxidant and immune system booster that protects against many forms of cancer. It repairs tissues, promotes healthy bones and teeth, lowers the risk of cancer, and alleviates acne and psoriasis. Retinol, the most active form of vitamin A, is used for cell renewal, wrinkle reduction, and collagen production.

vitamin b (panthenol b5)

This yellow oily acid, found widely in animal and vegetable foods, controls fat metabolism, is involved in energy production, and maintains healthy hair and skin. It also helps to counteract stress and boost metabolism. In skin care, vitamin B stimulates cells, aids in tissue repair, boosts the skin's moisture retention level, and holds water in products.

vitamin c (ascorbic acid)

Your immune system's best friend, this white crystalline vitamin present in plants, especially citrus fruits, tomatoes, and green vegetables, helps to fight infection and is an excellent antioxidant. In skin care, vitamin C slows the development of hyperpigmentation and age spots. It is necessary for healthy teeth, bones, skin, blood vessels, and collagen production.

vitamin c ester

This is a potent, fat-soluble form of vitamin C that gently and rapidly penetrates the skin. Vitamin C ester provides all the significant benefits of vitamin C (boosts collagen and elastin, resurfaces skin, and evens skin tone) and without any skin irritations, so it's excellent for more sensitive skin types.

vitamin e (tocopherol)

A superhero ingredient, vitamin E helps form red blood cells and muscle, and protects fat in the tissues from abnormal breakdown. Its antioxidant powers protect cells from damage and aid in wound healing. Vitamin E plays a crucial role in protecting skin cells and membranes from environmental damage. It also deeply moisturizes the skin, calms inflammation, and prevents irritation from sunburn. It's also an important preservative and antioxidant used to stabilize products against free radicals, prolonging a product's shelf life.

white tea

Like green tea, this wonder tea has high antioxidant levels due to its polyphenol and bioflavonoid content. Polyphenols are derived from the skin of red grapes, and bioflavonoids are found in fruits and vegetables.

willow extract

Produced from the willow tree, this mild astringent can be found in many infant-friendly products.

witch hazel

Witch hazel, derived from the leaves and bark of plants, is the go-to remedy for bug bites, bruises, and burns, due to its anti-inflammatory, anti-itching properties.

zinc oxide

Zinc oxide, a mineral derived from zinc, provides powerful protection from the UVA and UVB rays from the sun and is on the list of the FDA's approved sunscreens. It can sometimes produce a white color in products, but many times the particle size is reduced so it becomes transparent.

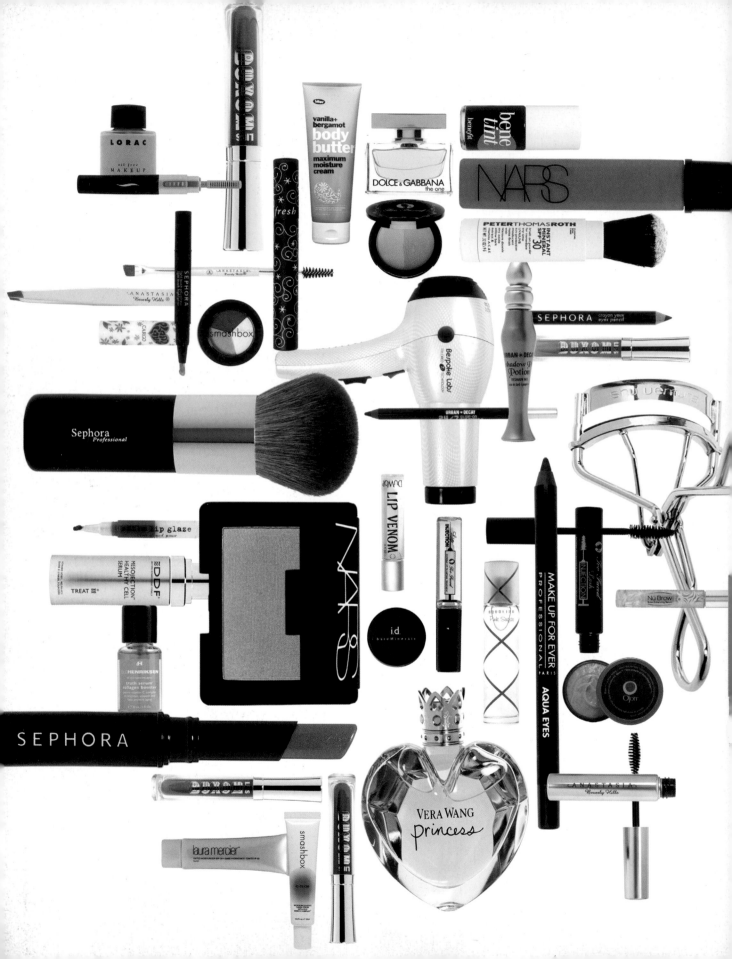

chapter 9

product
shopping
guide

SEPHORA'S 100 MUST-HAVES

If you could take a peek into the private cosmetic wardrobe of the savviest beauty addict around, it would look something like this list. We culled this shopping guide from the time-after-time bestselling products and the Sephora Best of Beauty Award Winners. We also asked our experts to name their personal favorites from their own brands and to tell us why they are so great. Whether you're just beginning to accrue your own signature beauty wardrobe, or you already have a cosmetics case full of long-ago-established staples, we bet you'll discover a brand-new life-changer from this list. Here, Sephora's 100 can't-live-without-'em products (in no particular order):

1. DIORSHOW UNLIMITED MASCARA IN BLACK:

The jumbo brush (originally designed for fashion show makeup artists to use on models) is like a magic wand for lashes—taking them from barely-there to bodacious.

2. THEBALM TIMEBALM CONCEALER:

"I won't walk out of the house without it. I have really dark circles and if I'm not wearing it, everyone thinks I didn't get any sleep," says Marissa Shipman, founder and CEO of TheBalm.

3. BARE ESCENTUALS BARE MINERALS FOUNDATION:

"If you're going to wear makeup every day of your life, then why not put something on your skin that will actually improve it? Our foundations contain exclusive, 100 percent pure bareMinerals without any preservatives, fillers, or binders—only the purest, highest quality minerals found in the earth," says Leslie Blodgett, CEO of Bare Escentuals.

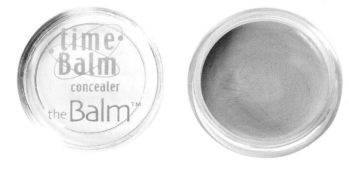

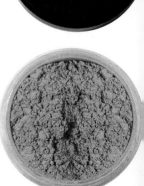

4. BENEFIT BENETINT: Originally invented as a nipple blush for a famous San Francisco stripper, this tiny bottle of ruby-tinted lip and cheek stain leaves a long-lasting rosy glow.

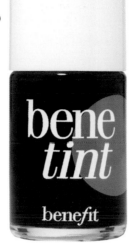

5. PETER THOMAS ROTH MINERAL POWDER SPF: "We were in the park with my kids on a cloudy, dark, fall afternoon when the sun came out. None of us, including my wife, were wearing any sunscreen (shame on us). I had my ultralight, oil-free SPF 30 sunblock on a string in my jacket pocket, but our hands were dirty from playing ball with the kids. That's when the idea struck me of coming out with a portable, nonmessy, easy-to-use, translucent SPF powder," says Peter Thomas Roth.

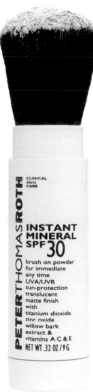

6. DDF MESOJECTION HEALTHY CELL SERUM: "I love this product because it's effective for all skin types/concerns and it contains a virtual patch technology that helps lock in hydration for hours. It also contains the next-generation antioxidants, scavenol and acai berry extract, so it should be used every day along with sunscreen to enhance free radical damage control," says DDF founder Dr. Howard Sobel.

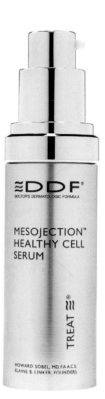

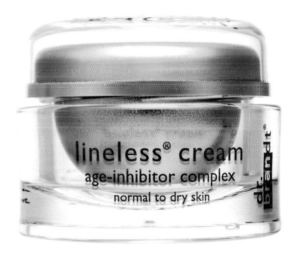

7. DR. BRANDT LINELESS CREAM: "All age groups can benefit from this because it helps preserve your elasticity, prevents collagen breakdown, and is a fabulous antioxidant," says Dr. Brandt.

8. N.V. PERRICONE M.D. FACE FIRMING ACTIVATOR: "This product really just does it all. It has ALA to minimize pores, DMAE to lift and tone the skin, and glycolic acid to resurface the skin. ALA also decreases scars, skin imperfections, discolorations, and uneven skin tone," says Dr. Perricone.

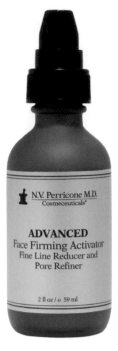

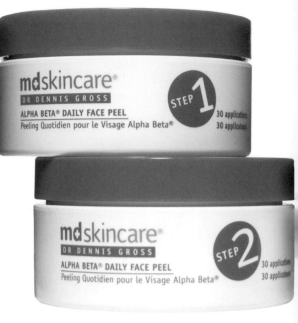

9. OLE HENRIKSEN TRUTH SERUM COLLAGEN BOOSTER: "It's lightweight, oil-free, and it instantly makes my skin glow with health and vitality. I easily look five years younger after it absorbs into my skin. It also delivers long-term results via a potent 10 percent antioxidant vitamin Ester-C complex that repairs damage and strengthens collagen. The real beauty of the formula is that it's so easy to use and can be applied right up under the eyes to firm this delicate area," says Ole Henriksen.

10. MD SKINCARE'S ALPHA BETA DAILY FACE PEEL: "It works to immediately improve the radiance and clarity of the skin and is unlike the harmful glycolic chemical peels of the early nineties. It improves skin density and firmness, diminishes fine lines and wrinkles, effectively treats acne and rosacea, helps prevent breakouts by regulating oil production, and helps skin achieve equilibrium, making oily skin less oily, and dry skin less dry," says Dr. Dennis Gross, creator of MD Skincare.

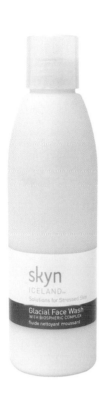

11. SKYN ICELAND GLACIAL FACE WASH: "I'm addicted to this product! I've always had problematic skin before starting this line, and now my skin has done a total 180. The first thing I do every morning and before I go to bed is use Glacial Face Wash. It's very concentrated so you only need a little bit. It's lathery, but won't strip your skin, and it's moisturizing but doesn't leave a film. And the scent is really clean and refreshing," says Sarah Kugelman, founder of Skyn Iceland.

13. ANTHONY LOGISTICS GLYCOLIC FACIAL WASH: "The first thing a guy should do is clean his face. Think of it this way: You would never wax your car without washing it first," says founder Tony Sosnick.

12. JUICE BEAUTY GREEN APPLE PEEL: "Every drop of this product really feeds your skin. After even one use, you'll see an immediate glow to the skin. There are over sixty organic ingredients added to the 100 percent organic apple, lemon, and grape juice base. Since crops can vary from season to season, the color of our products can be slightly different each time you buy them," says Karen Behnke, CEO of Juice Beauty.

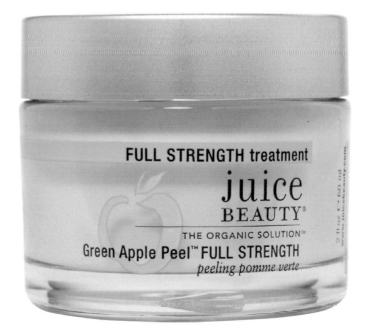

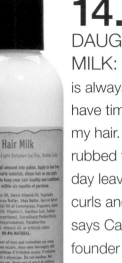

14. CAROL'S DAUGHTER HAIR MILK: "I am a person who is always on the go. I don't have time to spend styling my hair. A bit of Hair Milk rubbed through my hair every day leaves me with beautiful curls and no oily buildup," says Carol's Daughter founder Lisa Price.

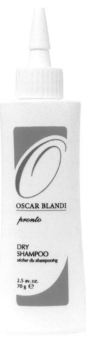

16. OSCAR BLANDI PRONTO DRY SHAMPOO: "You should only wash your hair two to three times a week because the follicles have a natural layer of protein that you'll strip if you overwash, and that's when dandruff builds up. Pronto cleans the scalp, gives the hair body and refreshes your follicles without washing," says Oscar Blandi.

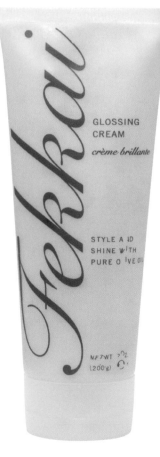

17. FRÉDÉRIC FEKKAI GLOSSING CREAM: "This is our core product! It adds shine to every hair type and is a great mixer with any other hair product," says Frédéric Fekkai.

15. FRESH SOY FACE CLEANSER: "It's extremely gentle and works on any skin type— you can even use it to remove eye makeup," says Fresh cofounder Lev Glazman.

18. MURAD DAILY RENEWAL COMPLEX: "Eat your vitamins and wear them, too! This formula contains high levels of vitamin C plus other antioxidants and skin soothers. It's patented and completely stable, which is a challenge when incorporating high levels of vitamin C, as it degrades and oxidizes when exposed to air or water, and Daily Renewal Complex contains zero water. It's proven, through independent studies, to reduce the appearance of photo-damage by 46 percent after four weeks of use," says Dr. Murad.

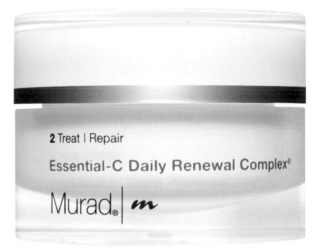

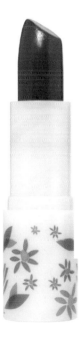

19. CARGO PLANT LOVE LIPSTICK: "This is a lipstick you can feel really good about. It's the first-ever lipstick tube made entirely out of corn, so it's compostable. The lipstick itself is petroleum-free, and the box is embedded with wildflower seeds, so you can plant it to grow," says Cargo founder Hana Zalzal.

20. TARTE CHEEK STAIN: "It's all-natural, features our patented t5 super fruit complex, and is so easy to use! Plus it gives cheeks the most healthy-looking flush," says Tarte founder Maureen Kelly.

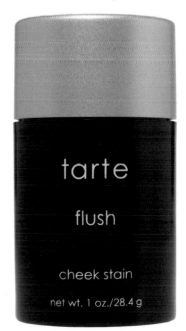

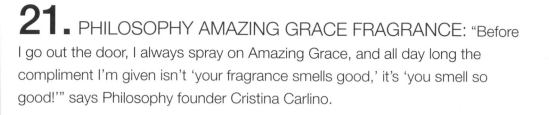

21. PHILOSOPHY AMAZING GRACE FRAGRANCE: "Before I go out the door, I always spray on Amazing Grace, and all day long the compliment I'm given isn't 'your fragrance smells good,' it's 'you smell so good!'" says Philosophy founder Cristina Carlino.

22. MAKE UP FOR EVER STAR POWDER: A shimmering, silky powder that literally looks good everywhere you apply it—on lips, eyes, cheeks, and décolletage.

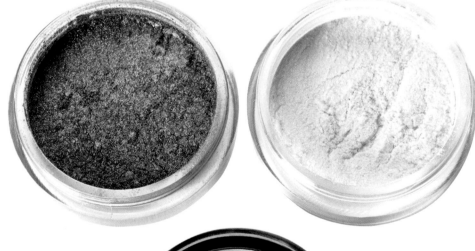

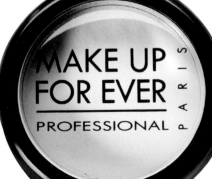

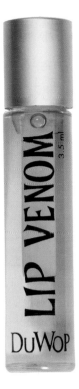

23. DUWOP LIP VENOM: For voluptuous lips faster than you can say "kiss me," Lip Venom is your secret weapon.

24. SUE DEVITT LUMINOUS FINISHING MIST: "You can transform any product into an anti-aging product with this mist, which gives you an immediate refreshed feeling," says Sue Devitt.

25. ANASTASIA HIGHLIGHTING PENCIL: "You can use this amazing pencil around the lips to make them look plumper, over a pimple to conceal It, and of course, under the brows for an immediate eye lift," says Anastasia Soare.

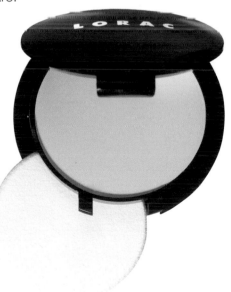

26. LORAC OIL FREE WET/DRY POWDER MAKEUP: "The silky, satiny texture of the powder makes the skin tone really smooth. It's fragrance-free so it's great for people like me with sensitive skin prone to breakouts," says LORAC founder Carol Shaw.

27. VINCENT LONGO AMERICANA LIPSTICK: "This sheer red color looks beautiful on everyone!" says Vincent Longo.

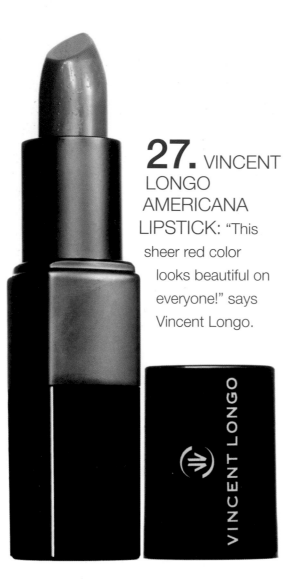

29. LAURA GELLER BRONZEN BRIGHTEN: "This is my desert-island product! It has six different hues, so you can pull them out separately and use one as an eyebrow fill-in color, and eyeliner, or an eye shadow," says Laura Geller.

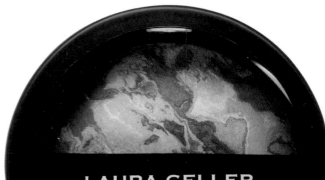

28. SHISEIDO MAKEUP ACCENTUATING COLOR STICK IN BRONZE: "Use this creamy stick before foundation to give the skin a glow—and you may not even need to apply much foundation," says makeup artist and Shiseido artistic director Dick Page.

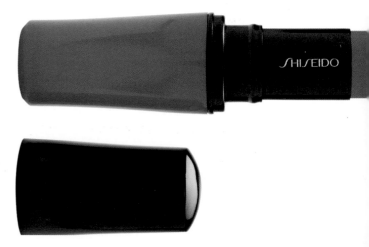

30. URBAN DECAY EYE SHADOW PRIMER POTION: Don't even attempt eye shadow without this nude primer. It acts like a magnet for shadow and liner, which means no creasing, running, or fading. You can literally take a shower with your eye makeup on and it will stay put.

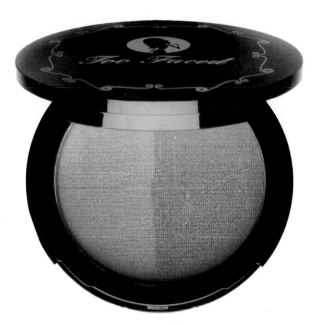

31. TOO FACED CARIBBEAN IN A COMPACT IN SUN BUNNY: "Tan skin looks healthier, younger, and sexier, but NEVER sacrifice your health for beauty! And you don't have to with Sun Bunny—half has a pink undertone and the other half has a traditional bronze undertone, so when you mix them together you get a perfectly real-looking tan!" says Too Faced founder Jerrod Blandino.

32. URBAN DECAY MIDNIGHT COWBOY: This beige shadow flecked with silver glitter is loaded with pigments, which makes eyes—no matter what their color—pop.

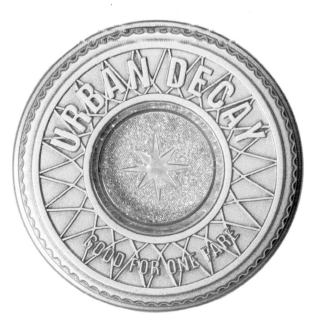

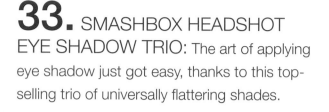

33. SMASHBOX HEADSHOT EYE SHADOW TRIO: The art of applying eye shadow just got easy, thanks to this top-selling trio of universally flattering shades.

34. SEPHORA COLORFUL EYE SHADOW PALETTE IN KISS: A must-have for your office drawer—the rich bronze/gold shades take you from subtle and shimmery for day to all-out gilded gorgeousness for night.

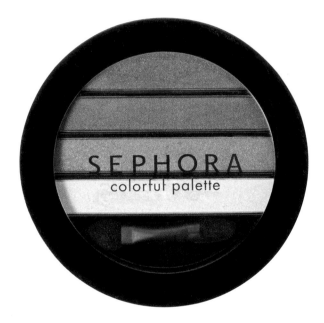

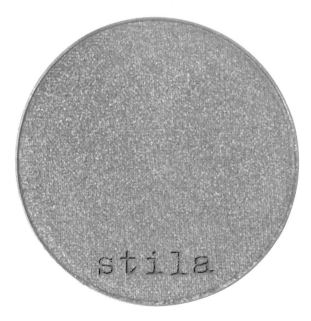

35. STILA EYE SHADOW IN KITTEN: This shimmering nude is a must for every makeup wardrobe. Wear alone or use it as a base for a sultry smoky eye.

36. SMASHBOX PHOTO FINISH FOUNDATION PRIMER: "Every great makeup application begins with the perfect canvas. Photo Finish smoothes and perfects the skin while extending makeup wear for an all-day flawless finish," says Smashbox cofounder Dean Factor.

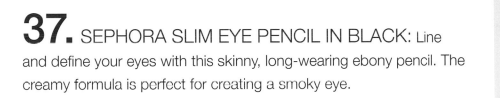

37. SEPHORA SLIM EYE PENCIL IN BLACK: Line and define your eyes with this skinny, long-wearing ebony pencil. The creamy formula is perfect for creating a smoky eye.

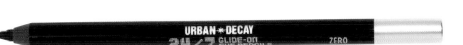

38. URBAN DECAY 24/7 GLIDE ON PENCIL IN ZERO: Just like the name says, this budge-proof liner sticks around all day, and with its ultraluxe, moisturizing formula, you'll be glad that it does.

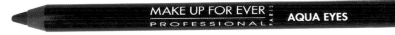

39. MAKE UP FOR EVER AQUA EYES EYELINER IN BLACK: A wedding-day essential due to its ability to withstand sweat, tears, and countless flashbulbs.

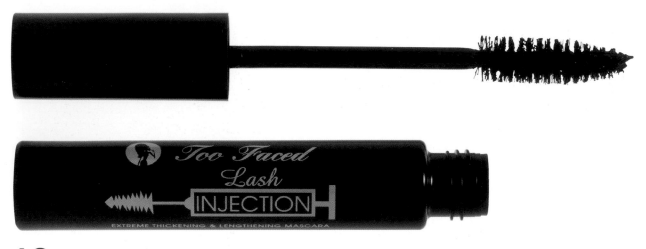

40. TOO FACED LASH INJECTION: Expect the same massive swelling that Too Faced's beloved Lip Injection does for lips, but this time on your lashes. The breakthrough formula literally forms tubes around each lash, extending way past the tips to create major volume and length.

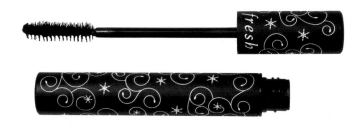

42. LANCÔME HYPNOSE MASCARA IN DEEP BLACK: "We're the world leader in luxury mascara, so our mascaras really deliver. This one, without a doubt, gives you thick, extended lashes that are the blackest color possible," says Ross Burton, Lancôme's national artistic director.

41. FRESH SUPERNOVA MASCARA IN BLACK: This conditioning mascara enriched with panthenol, protective linden extract, and nourishing meadowfoam oil thickens, extends, and delivers an ultraglossy finish in one coat.

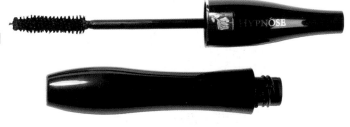

43. NARS BLUSH ORGASM:
The reigning candidate for the perfect shade of blush, this peachy-pink shade with a slight hint of shimmer makes everyone glow like they just . . . well, you know . . .

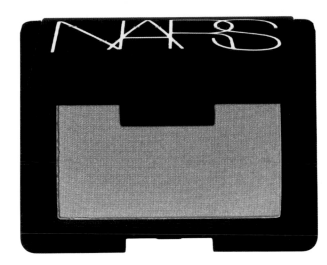

44. SEPHORA LUMINOUS TRIP
IN ROSE: Buff this palette of three glowing shades of shimmer over cheeks, eyes, shoulders and décolletage—anywhere you want your skin to sparkle.

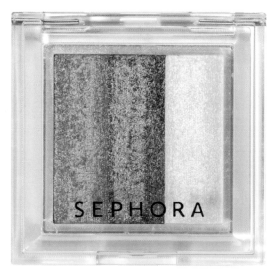

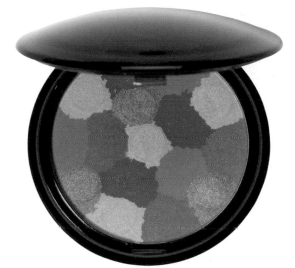

45. GUERLAIN TERRACOTTA LIGHT SHEER BRONZING POWDER
IN BRUNETTE: Terracotta has set the benchmark for the natural, sun-kissed look since 1984. The oil-absorbing powder's still our fave for the perfectly real-looking faux glow.

46. SMASHBOX
O GLOW: When you apply this intuitive gel blush, your skin's moisture activates the energizing Goji Berry-C Complex, creating a microcirculatory effect. The result? The exact shade you naturally blush.

47. LAURA MERCIER TINTED MOISTURIZER: For those who can get away with minimal coverage, this sheer, sunscreen-infused tint leaves skin fresh and dewy.

49. STILA SHEER TINTED MOISTURIZER: Packed with sun protection and just enough color to even skin tone, this light, hydrating formula is ideal for all skin types and comes in natural, see-through shades.

48. BENEFIT YOU REBEL: This much-loved tinted moisturizer is a travel must—it provides light coverage, moisture, and sun protection.

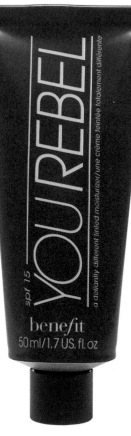

50. SEPHORA LIGHT TOUCH HIGHLIGHTER: This light, creamy highlighting pen banishes brown spots, shadows, and dark circles, brightening and refreshing the contours of your face.

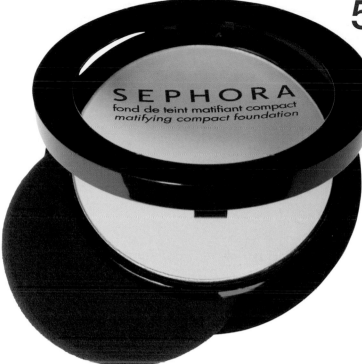

51. SEPHORA MATTIFYING COMPACT FOUNDATION:

This feather-light pressed powder foundation glides on, leaving a poreless, porcelain-like finish. Each supernatural shade can be applied wet or dry, depending on the coverage you desire.

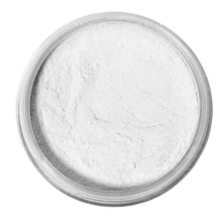

52. BARE ESCENTUALS MINERAL VEIL: For

the ultimate translucent finishing touch, this powder melts into skin, infusing it with light, putting your look into soft focus.

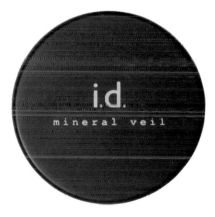

53. NARS LIP GLOSS IN ORGASM: A spin-off of their bestselling blush,

Nars introduced this golden pink lip gloss to many excited fans.

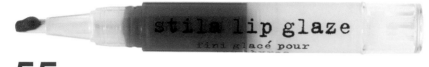

54. SEPHORA MANIAC LONG WEARING LIPSTICK IN 08: A highly
pigmented, long-lasting lipstick. This rich shade of bronze glides on smooth with an intense, stay-true color that lasts all day—and night.

55. STILA LIP GLAZE IN SUGAR: The click-and-glaze brush allows pro-quality application and the sheer, ultra-shiny formula keeps your lips glossier, longer.

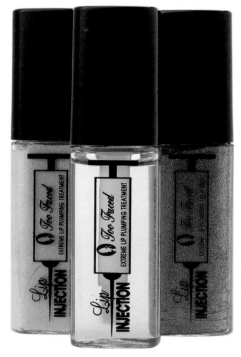

56. BARE ESCENTUALS BUXOM LIPS IN AMBER: Infused with sparkling minerals and the plumping power of peptides (which stimulate collagen over time), this gloss leaves lips seriously full-bodied.

57. TOO FACED LIP INJECTION: This tingly treatment, which employs vitamin B and capsium Chinese extract, boosts circulation in lips, plumping them up to a new level of lusciousness.

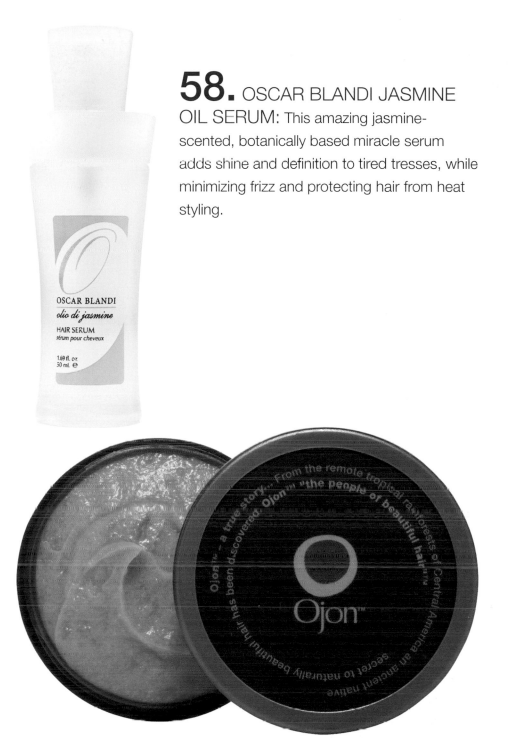

58. OSCAR BLANDI JASMINE OIL SERUM: This amazing jasmine-scented, botanically based miracle serum adds shine and definition to tired tresses, while minimizing frizz and protecting hair from heat styling.

59. OJON RESTORATIVE TREATMENT: This intensive hair rejuvenator contains 100 percent Ojon palm nut oil to improve damaged, color-treated, or processed hair without weighing it down.

60. ANASTASIA ALL ABOUT BROWS KIT IN ASH BLOND: Almost as good as scoring an appointment with Anastasia herself, this six-piece kit has all the specialized tools you need to get perfect arches.

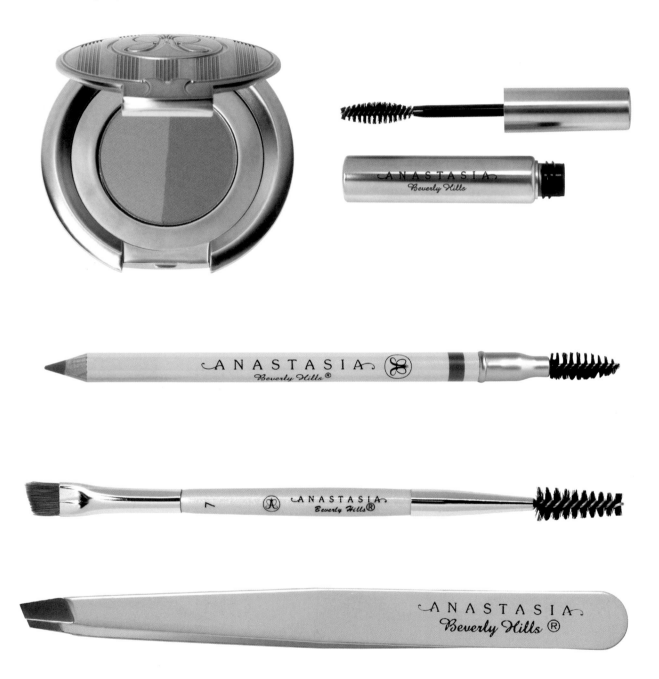

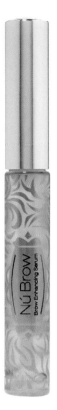

61. ANASTASIA NÚ BROW ENHANCING SERUM:
The overly tweezed can take comfort in this treatment that improves brow fullness. Capilectine stimulates the hair follicle and capigen helps prolong the hair's growth phase.

64. COSMEDICINE MEDI-MATTE OIL CONTROL LOTION SUNSCREEN SPF 20:
Say good-bye to oil slicks and hello to this antioxidant and SPF-packed lotion that keeps skin shine-free for up to

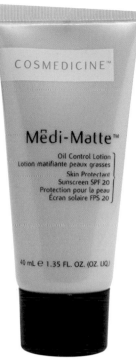

62. LORAC CREAMY BROW PENCIL:
A makeup bag must: This multitasking formula colors, fills in, defines, and shapes brows subtly, while the spooly brush grooms unruly hairs.

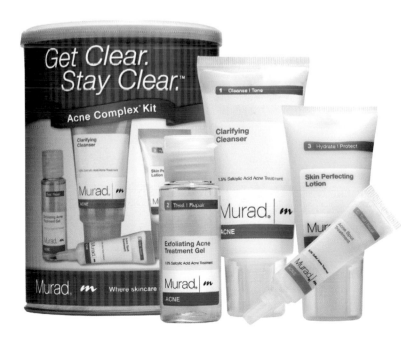

63. MURAD ACNE COMPLEX STARTER KIT:
Introduce yourself to Dr. Murad's acne-fighting regimen, with minis of his top clear-skin treatments.

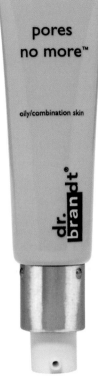

65. DR. BRANDT PORES NO MORE:
This classic pore patroller packs antibacterial tea tree to nix breakouts and oil-absorbing microspheres to mattify skin and disguise pores.

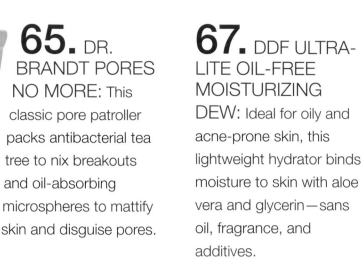

67. DDF ULTRA-LITE OIL-FREE MOISTURIZING DEW:
Ideal for oily and acne-prone skin, this lightweight hydrator binds moisture to skin with aloe vera and glycerin—sans oil, fragrance, and additives.

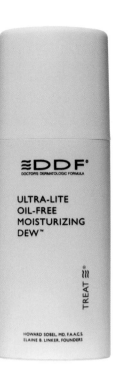

66. KINERASE CREAM:
This gentle cream nurses dry skin and—thanks to kinetin, a powerful-but-gentle antioxidant—improves fine lines, wrinkles, and sun damage.

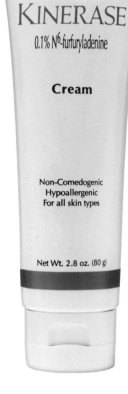

68. BLISS THE YOUTH AS WE KNOW IT:
This extraordinary cream—made with Bliss's ten most effective age-fighting ingredients—is a one-stop shop for skin regeneration.

69. PHILOSOPHY HOPE IN A JAR:
Year after year, award after award, this standout radiance-boosting moisturizer delivers antioxidants and lactic acid to exfoliate and brighten skin.

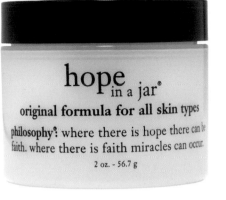

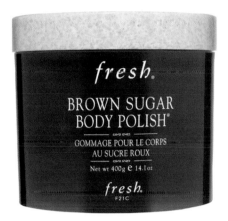

70. FRESH BROWN SUGAR BODY POLISH:
This bestselling mix of real brown sugar crystals and healing oils has an instant brightening, softening effect on skin.

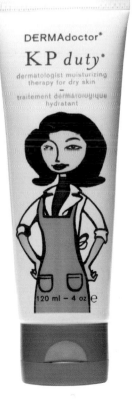

71. DERMADOCTOR KP DUTY:
A dermatologist favorite, this unique product controls keratosis pilaris (aka chicken skin) with smoothing glycolic acid and urea.

72. CAROL'S DAUGHTER ALMOND COOKIE SHEA SOUFFLÉ:
An addictively light and fluffy soufflé made with all-natural almond, vanilla, and sandalwood.

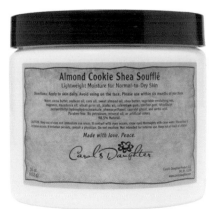

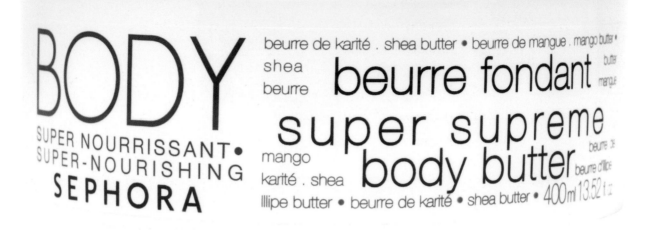

73. SEPHORA SUPER SUPREME
BODY BUTTER: A decadently rich body
butter that uses shea butter to pamper,
moisturize, nourish, and protect.

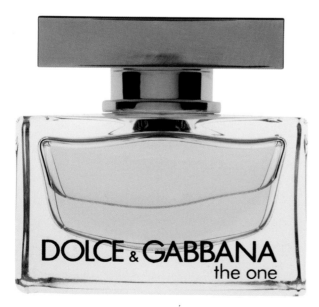

74. DOLCE & GABBANA THE
ONE: This warm Oriental incorporates fruity
notes of bergamot and mandarin, as well as
lychee and peach.

75. EMPORIO ARMANI DIAMONDS: An unexpectedly gourmand floral fragrance with a heart of rose, blended with luscious lychee, cedar wood, and amber.

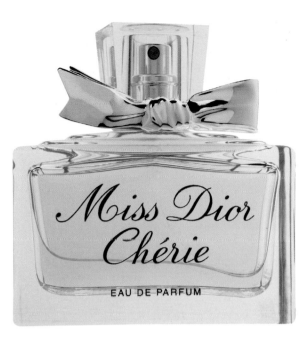

76. MISS DIOR CHÉRIE: This blend of tangerine, strawberry leaves, and caramelized popcorn is a slightly sweeter take on the original Miss Dior from 1947.

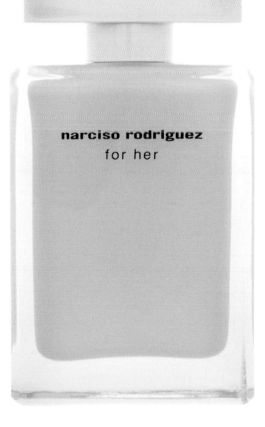

77. NARCISO RODRIGUEZ: A fashionable blend of pink chypre and pink flowers, warmed with Egyptian musk, amber, and flower honey.

78. DAISY BY MARC JACOBS:
Girly and sophisticated all at once, this
bouquet of violet leaves, wild strawberries,
and violet petals is sure to please every Marc
Jacobs devotee.

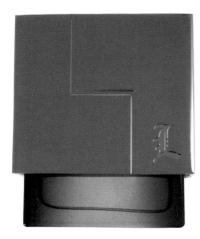

79. LAMB BY GWEN
STEFANI: With notes of sparkling
green, leafy water hyacinth, pear, and
heliotrope flower, it fuses feminine florals
with masculine musks. This scent is as
edgy as Gwen herself.

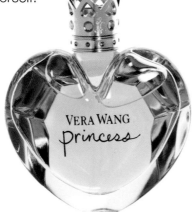

80. VERA WANG PRINCESS:
Edgy with effortless style, this royally gorgeous
scent is an exotic fruity floral bouquet with a
twist of pink guava and vanilla.

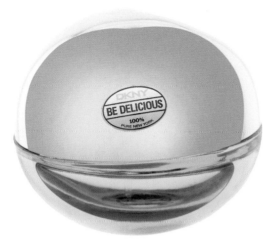

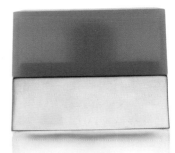

83. DOLCE & GABBANA LIGHT BLUE: A vivacious fragrance that blends Sicilian citron, Granny Smith apple, bluebells, and white rose.

81. DKNY BE DELICIOUS: A fresh-picked blend of apple, cucumber, tuberose, and white amber.

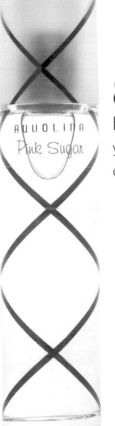

82. BLISS VANILLA + BERGAMOT BODY BUTTER: For skin that's smooth as buttah but never greasy, slather on this heaven-scented mix of vanilla, amber, lemon, bergamot, myrrh, and musk. It's easy to become addicted to the silky soft and mouth-wateringly moist feeling you get after each application.

84. AQUOLINA PINK SUGAR: A fun, youthful scent of cotton candy and vanilla.

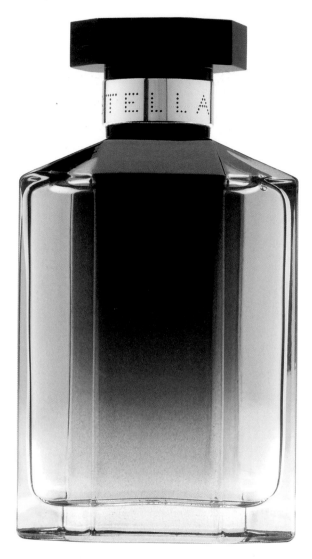

85. STELLA MCCARTNEY STELLA: This sophisticated scent pairs the playfulness of rose and peony with the darker appeal of amber.

86. JUICY COUTURE SCOTTY: A playful blend of watermelon, wild rose, marigold, and caramel crème brûlée.

87. YVES SAINT LAURENT L'HOMME: A sparkling combination of bergamot, ginger, and vetiver, plus magnetic notes of basil flower, white pepper, and tonka bean.

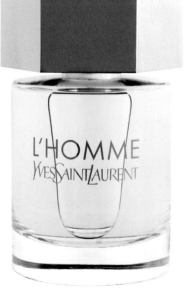

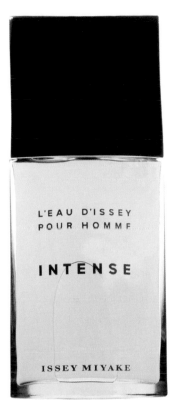

88. ISSEY MIYAKE L'EAU D'ISSEY POUR HOMME INTENSE: Like the original, captivating L'Eau D'Issey Pour Homme, the fragrance has a heart of mandarin orange zest, but this version is enhanced with warmer notes of cardamom, cinnamon, nutmeg, and papyrus wood.

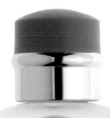

89. DOLCE & GABBANA LIGHT BLUE POUR HOMME: A nod to D&G's native Italy, this scent captures the Mediterranean's sensuality. Frozen grapefruit peel, Szechuan pepper, and oak create a blend that's woody and spicy.

90. PRADA AMBER POUR HOMME: This stylish scent—a masculine mélange of musk, sandalwood, orange blossom, and tonka bean—is tasteful and timeless.

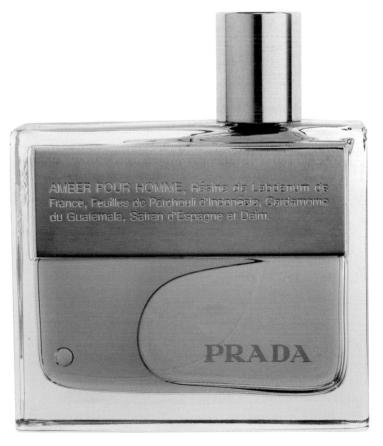

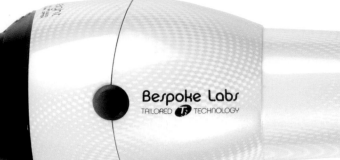

91. T3 BESPOKE LABS FEATHERWEIGHT DRYER: A true beauty phenomenon, this high-tech dryer is infused with tourmaline—a semiprecious stone that emits far-infrared heat to dry hair 60 percent faster.

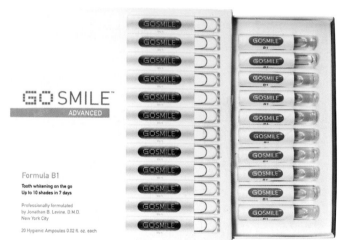

93. GOSMILE ADVANCED FORMULA B1 TOOTH WHITENING ON THE GO: When you can't brush your teeth between meals, go straight to GoSmile. Clinically proven to whiten teeth four to ten shades in seven days (depending on your starting shade), this high-speed whitening system is packed in sleek, vacuum-sealed portable ampoules for easy use, anywhere.

92. SEPHORA MINI HEATED EYELASH CURLER: This lash innovation is perfect for curling stubborn straight lashes. Simply turn on, wait fifteen seconds, and use it as you would a mascara brush.

94. NARS LIPSTICK IN DOLCE VITA: This universally flattering neutral has a sheer dusty rose hue that works for day *and* night.

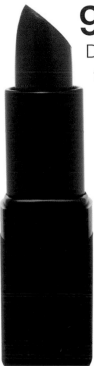
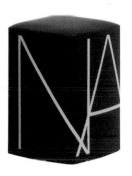

96. LANCÔME FLASH BRONZER GLOW 'N WEAR: This quick-drying gel wins our vote for the biggest faker. It leaves skin with a naturally tawny glow sans any transference onto clothing or hair.

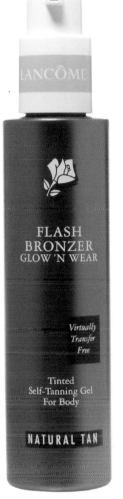

FLASH BRONZER GLOW 'N WEAR

Virtually Transfer Free

Tinted Self-Tanning Gel For Body

NATURAL TAN

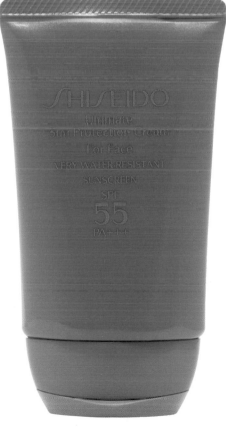

95. SHISEIDO ULTIMATE SUN PROTECTION CREAM SPF 55: Goes on like butter, leaving no visible white residue or trace of stickiness; it also contains antioxidants and the retexturizing ingredient Xylitol to counteract roughness and keep skin looking soft and healthy.

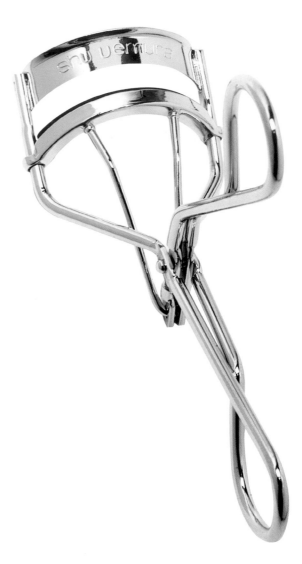

98. SHU UEMURA EYELASH CURLER: Look in every top makeup artist's kit and undoubtedly you'll find this eyelash curler. It has the power to transform your entire look in seconds. Some beauties even stock up on three or more to keep at the office, home and on the go.

97. SEPHORA BRONZER BRUSH: This Best of Sephora winner makes bronzing easy. Get a flawless application every time thanks to the jumbo thicket of high-grade goat hair.

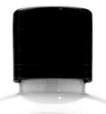

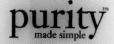

99. PHILOSOPHY PURITY MADE SIMPLE: Use this beloved cleanser to remove makeup and get skin squeaky clean. It's even gentle enough to use as a lingerie wash!

philosophy®: purity is natural. we come into this world with all the right instincts. we are innocent, and therefore perceive things as they should be, rather than how they are. our conscience is clear, our hands are clean, and the world at large is truly beautiful. it is at this time we feel most blessed. to begin feeling young again, we must begin with the most basic step of all; the daily ritual of cleansing.

one-step facial cleanser
16 fl. oz. - 473.1 ml

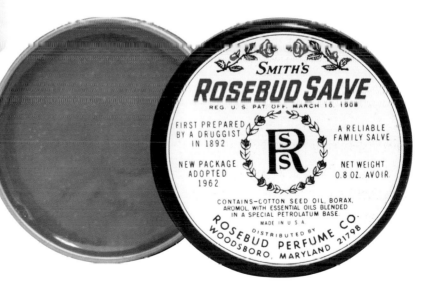

100. SMITH'S ROSEBUD SALVE: A cult favorite, multipurpose lip balm that soothes dry lips and leaves a slightly glossy, perfectly kissable sheen atop bare lips and lipstick.

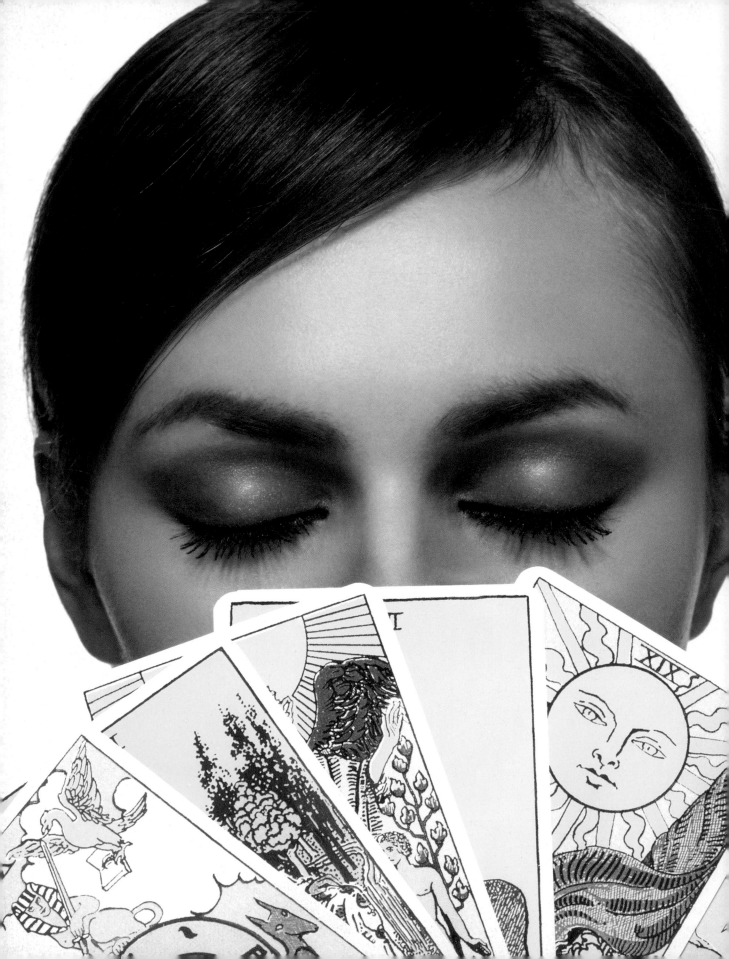

the future of beauty

What does the future have in store for our health, appearance, and well-being?
The experts take a peek at their crystal balls. Here, their predictions . . .

"In the future, I think we're going to see a merging of the health care system and the beauty industry. By merging the two, people will understand that staying beautiful is really about staying healthy. I do not believe that the future lies in an acceleration of invasive treatments, injectible fillers, neurotoxins, or radical surgery. Great breakthroughs are being made that introduce safe, yet genuinely transformative methodologies that not only help restore damaged, aging skin to youthful suppleness, but reinvigorate the entire body."
—Dr. Perricone

"There's always been an emphasis on beauty—throughout history and in every culture. Just look how beauty has been—and still is—worshipped with rituals. As we move forward into the future, there will be a continued appreciation for beauty. Technology will continue to advance, allowing us to use the best and purest ingredients while the emphasis on the natural will increase, especially with the renewed awareness we have for the well-being of our planet." **—Ole Henriksen**

"The future of beauty is the redefinition of what is beautiful without racial boundaries or parameters. Face-lifts without surgery. Natural and organic without being 'crunchy.' Beautiful formulas, textures, and packages that are good for you and the environment. Ingestibles that make us healthy, rid us of acne, eradicate the signs of aging, and dissolve fat."

—Sarah Kugelman, Skyn Iceland

"Soon we'll be able to regenerate different parts of the body with the use of stem cells. For example, if you don't like the color or shape of your eyes, you'd be able to replace them with bigger, bluer ones. You'll even be able to alter the shape of your nose. Stem cell technology will allow you to put on a new layer of skin, where old skin has been damaged. That's the future!"

—Dr. Howard Murad

"Organic beauty is growing at 20 percent a year, so the future certainly holds more organic offerings. I can envision people having a mini cosmetic refrigerator in the bathroom to hold products that are really fresh. I can also see people demanding more customization and adding boosters to products."

—Karen Behnke, Juice Beauty

"The future of beauty is green. We're going to see an interesting combination of efficiency and recyclability, but companies will still try and find a way to keep the glamour and luxury in the product. Just like a lot of car companies are introducing hybrids, beauty companies will come out with second lines that are environmentally friendly."

—Lisa Price, Carol's Daughter

"Over time we'll see the ability to forecast and visualize what people could look like in a three-dimensional format. People will be able to preview what they might look like if they plump their lips, lengthen their teeth, or use a certain beauty product. This will help people to make a decision about what path to take to look the way they want."

—Dr. Jonathan Levine, GoSmile

"Taking the time out of your day to visit a salon every time you need a cut and color, or even taking a shower with running water to wash and condition your hair, will be almost as archaic as the busy signal on a rotary dial phone. Tress Tablets will be available in a variety of formulas, which are customized by your stylist to offer you the luxury of controlling and changing your hair's style, length, and color on a whim."

—Oscar Blandi

"We're working on developing a product that will correct or change the texture of your hair. If your hair is curly, it will make it straight; if you have thin hair, this will make it thicker."

—Frédéric Fekkai

"Imagine a blush that peels off like a second skin and can be worn for days at a time. Or an eyeliner that mimics tattoo or henna drawing and lasts for a week. The old-style stains for cheeks and lips will turn into sheerer washes of semipermanent color that are easier to work with and will offer a natural, longer-lasting finish. These products will also be good for the skin, plumping and firming as they are applied."

—Hana Zalzal, Cargo

"I think the natural trend is here to stay! It's all about having healthy ingredients in your beauty products. Fruit extracts, preservative- and paraben-free products are definitely playing an important role."

—Mauren Kelly, Tarte

"More and more beauty companies are branching away from marketing to a simple demographic (i.e., 18–34, 45–60). The same way the world is getting smaller as technology grows, we're becoming a more global community, and women of all ages are enjoying the same beauty products. A hip grandmother and her tween granddaughter are starting to buy the same makeup and skin care."

—Cristina Bartolucci, DuWop

"I think a lot of the classic formulas we've seen will be revamped and reworked. I also think whitening products for the skin will be huge— to correct sun damage, redness, and rashes. Formulas will become cleaner, with new active ingredients that are more organic in nature."

—Vincent Longo

"With the ever-growing concern about our environment, consumers are tuned in to sustainable packaging. When their favorite fragrance needs to be replenished, how nice would it be if they could go to their favorite retail location to get the bottle refilled, or perhaps just return the empty bottle so that it could be recycled?"

—Mary Ellen Lapsansky, executive director of the Fragrance Foundation

"In the future, there will be products that make the skin look even more perfect, especially for technology like high-definition television, where even the smallest flaw can show. To that end, we're creating a line of high-definition makeup!"

—Dany Sanz, creator of Make Up For Ever

"I firmly believe that the topical application of vitamins (applied directly to the skin) and the increased effort to combat environmental aggressors, prevent aging, and treat existing skin conditions are the top trends in skin care. In fact, a mathematical analysis shows that a 2 percent Vitamin C gel applied directly to the face is 200 times more potent than consuming a 600 milligram Vitamin C pill! Applying ingredients to our skin early on can make a significant difference in preventing premature aging."

—Dr. Dennis Gross, MD Skincare

"Consumers will move away from the department stores and shop online and in open-sell environments where there's less pressure and it's a lot more fun to shop."

—Dean Factor, Smashbox

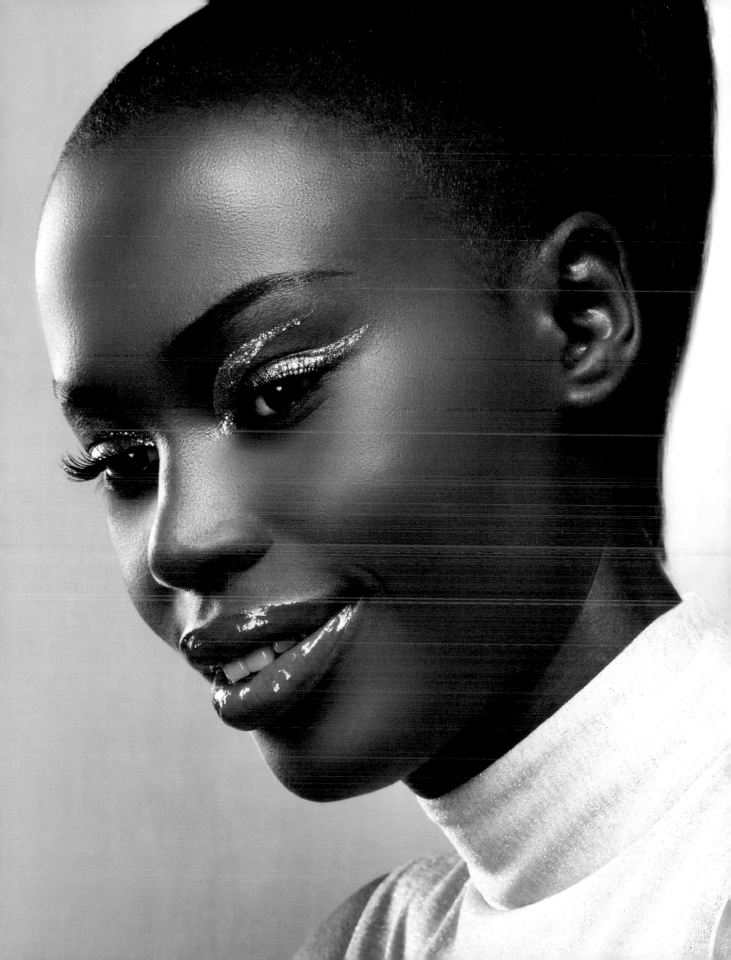

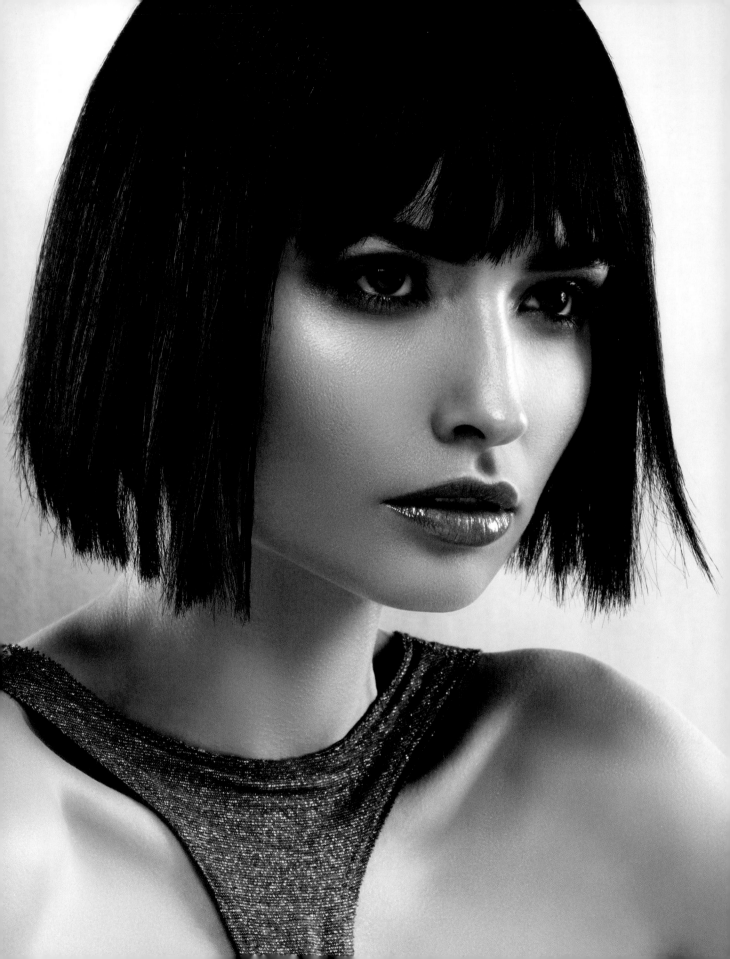

"*As the public becomes more and more educated through the Internet and television, their demands will only continue to become more extreme. We will be able to give people with unrealistic expectations the results they've been dreaming of: mascaras that actually grow hair; foundations and powders that lift and firm the skin; body lotions that eliminate cellulite. Surgery won't be as prevalent because we're going to be able to offer many of the same results with our cosmetics.*"

—Jerrod Blandino, Too Faced

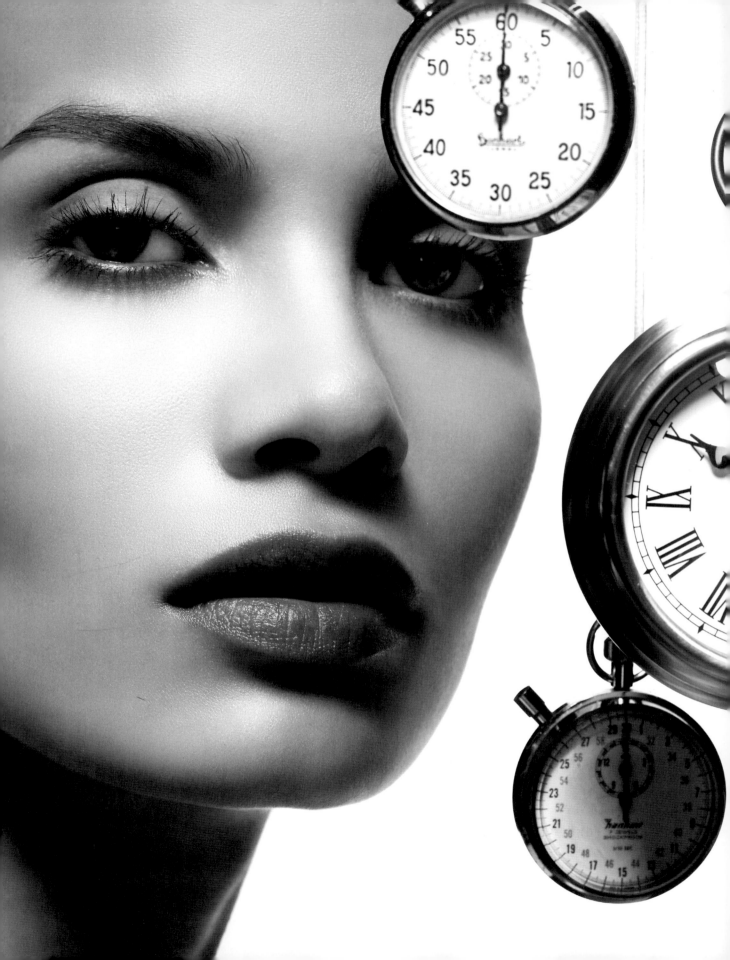

APPENDIX A: TIMING IS EVERYTHING

As with food, beauty products can go bad, too. Depending on their ingredients, cosmetics can spoil or simply lose their potency. Thanks to new labeling on some products (an open-jar icon, with the number of months it's good for after opening), it is becoming easier to figure out cosmetic expiration dates. But for unlabeled beauty loot, use this tossing schedule to guide you.

one year

blush: Cheek color (creams and powders) should be replaced yearly. However, washing your blush brush every few weeks will help keep it bacteria-free.

eau de parfum: Most fragrances are good for one year if you use them two times per week and store them in a cool, dark place. Sprays retain their scent longer than splashes, which tend to turn more quickly because they're exposed to air every time you remove the cap.

SPF: Although technically sunscreen is good for a year from the day you buy it, after a summer spent sitting out in the sun or stashed in a steamy, hot beach bag, your SPF is pretty much shot. The sun-blocking chemicals in the lotion lose their oomph and can become ineffective. Replace every season.

six months

facial moisturizer: Creams that contain antioxidants are very sensitive to light and expire quickly, especially ones with vitamins A, C, and E. Products with acids like glycolic, salicylic, and beta hydroxy will last the longest.

eye makeup: Your eyes are extra prone to bacterial infection, so anything touching them— cream and powder shadows, liners—should be tossed after six months.

three months

mascara: Since it's extremely prone to microbial growth (the wand pushes air and bacteria into the tube), play it safe and replace your mascara at least every three months.

concealer: Because it is used every day and (depending on its dispenser) is usually in contact with the air for long amounts of time, concealer should be replaced regularly. Be sure to wash your concealer brush frequently, and, if you use your fingers to apply, always wash your hands first.

liquid foundation: Foundation packed in wide-mouthed jars should be tossed at three months since the jars expose the makeup to greater amounts of air, upping the chances of bacterial growth.

APPENDIX B: SEPHORA MASTERS

Cristina Bartolucci, cofounder and creative director of DuWop Cosmetics

Gina Bertolotti, senior stylist at the Oscar Blandi Salon in New York City

Karen Behnke, CEO of Juice Beauty

Oscar Blandi, founder of Oscar Blandi Hair Care and owner of the Oscar Blandi Salon

Jerrod Blandino, founder and creative director of Too Faced

Leslie Blodgett, CEO of Bare Escentuals

Fredric Brandt, MD, Miami and New York City dermatologist and founder of Dr. Brandt Skincare

Ross Burton, national artistic director at Lancôme

Cristina Carlino, founder and CEO of philosophy

Anne Marie Cilmi, director of development and education at Bliss

Sean Combs, fashion designer, musician, and founder of Sean Jean fragrances

Sue Devitt, makeup artist and founder of Sue Devitt Studio

Davis Factor, photographer and cofounder and CCO of Smashbox

Dean Factor, cofounder and CEO of Smashbox

Jane Ford, cofounder of Benefit Cosmetics

Jean Ford, cofounder of Benefit Cosmetics

Frédéric Fekkai, founder of Fekkai Hair Care and owner of Frédéric Fekkai salons

Laura Geller, founder of Laura Geller Makeup

Lev Glazman, cofounder and president of research and development at Fresh

Dr. Dennis Gross, dermatologist and creator of MD Skincare

Ole Henriksen, founder of Ole Henriksen Skin Care, owner of Ole Henriksen Spa in Los Angeles

Victoria Jackson, celebrity makeup artist

Maureen Kelly, founder and CEO of Tarte

Sarah Kugelman, president and founder of Skyn ICELAND

Mary Ellen Lapsansky, executive director of The Fragrance Foundation

Dr. Jonathan Levine, prosthodontist and founder of Go Smile

Vincent Longo, makeup artist and founder of Vincent Longo

Howard Murad, MD, FAAD, associate clinical professor of medicine at UCLA; CEO and founder of Murad, Inc.

Dick Page, makeup artist and artistic director for Shiseido The Makeup

Shane Paish, Dior global makeup advisor

Dr. Nicholas Perricone, MD, FACN, founder and CEO of NV Perricone MD. Ltd.

Lisa Price, founder of Carol's Daughter

Peter Thomas Roth, CEO of Peter Thomas Roth Labs

Dany Sanz, founder of Make Up For Ever

Carol Shaw, makeup artist and founder of LORAC

Randi Shinder, CEO and founder, Fusion Beauty, Clean Perfume, Dessert Beauty

Marissa Shipman, founder of theBalm

Melissa Silver, makeup artist for Bourjois

Anastasia Soare, brow specialist and founder of Anastasia Beverly Hills

Dr. Howard Sobel, dermatologist, founder of DDF skincare

Gilbert Soliz, Sephora Pro Beauty Team member

Tony Sosnick, founder of Anthony Logistics

Kyle White, senior colorist at the Oscar Blandi Salon in New York City

Hana Zalzal, founder and president of CARGO

Wende Zomnir, cocreator and creative director of Urban Decay

ACKNOWLEDGMENTS

This book could not have been possible without the support, encouragement, and hard work of all the beautiful, talented people at Sephora, Trident Media Group, and HarperCollins. A big thanks to David Suliteanu, Allison Slater, Jessica Stacey, Corinne de Ocejo, Abbie Pearlstein, Susannah Davis, Jon Hymowitz, Heather Gray, Laura Kenney, Tamie Segal, Cindy Fedida, Mary Ellen O'Neill, Cassandra Gonzalez, Lorie Pagnozzi, Amy Vreeland, Shelby Meizlik, Jean Marie Kelly, Darryl Patterson, Nick Baratta, and Amy Meyerson.

A very special thanks to Kathy Huck at Collins for understanding and staying true to the vision. To Eileen Cope at Trident, who saw the potential for this book from the get-go and tirelessly went above and beyond to make it happen. To Elizabeth Lippman for always bringing out my best smile. To the inspirational Betsy Olum for her infectious enthusiasm and careful guidance. To the incomparable Bernadette Fitzpatrick for her amazing creative direction and wicked senses of style and humor. A heartfelt thank-you to Alice, Bruce, and Eric Schweiger, my personal cheering section.

photo credits

Pages *vi*, 2, 3 (top), 6, 15 (top), 16, 17 (top), 20–21, 22, 27 (right and bottom), 28, 32, 35, 39, 40, 41, 42, 49, 50 (all), 52, 57, 58, 60, 64, 65 (left and middle), 66, 68, 71, 77, 82, 88, 96, 207 courtesy of Fernando Milani; pp. *viii*, 8, 26, 27 (top left), 29, 34, 92, 95 courtesy of Karina Taira; pp. *x*, 44, 61, 72, 73, 76, 198 courtesy of Donna Trope; p. 3 (bottom) courtesy of Frédéric Fekkai; p. 4 (left) courtesy of Cristina Carlino; pp. 4 (right top), 18 courtesy of Josie Lepe; p. 4 (right bottom) courtesy of Laura Geller; p. 5 (left) courtesy of Lancôme; p. 5 (right) courtesy of Dick Page; p. 11 (middle) courtesy of courtesy of Clarins; pp. 11 (top and bottom), 12, 13, 14, 19, 25, 33, 37, 46, 47, 48, 53, 59, 62, 63, 67, 74, 75, 79, 83, 91 (top), 99, 100, 139, 146–147 (middle), 154, 155 (top), 156, 158, 159, 160 (top), 166–197, 201 courtesy of Darryl Patterson; pp. 15 (bottom), 54, 80, 84, 85 (top and middle), 114 (photos of Oscar Blandi and Dr. Perricone), 146 (left), 152 courtesy of Phillipe Salomon; p. 17 (bottom) courtesy of Aimee Herring; pp. 24, 137 (bottom), 164, 102–112 courtesy of Sephora; pp. 30, 36, 65 (right), 200, 203, 204 courtesy of Cleo Sullivan; p. 31 courtesy of Randi Shinder; p. 45 courtesy of Sarah Sloboda; p. 55, 56, 114 (photo of Maureen Kelly), 135, 136, 137 (top), 142, 145 courtesy of Elizabeth Lipmann; p. 78 (bottom) © iStockphoto/LongHa2006; p. 78 (top) © iStockphoto/sorsillo; p. 78 (middle) © iStockphoto/joxxxxjo; p. 81, 85 (bottom) courtesy of Ralf Nau/Getty Images: p. 87 © iStockphoto/niDerLander; p. 91 (bottom) © iStockphoto/parisassoc; p. 114 (photo of Jarrod Blandino) courtesy Jarrod Blandino; pp. 114 (photos of Gilbert Soliz and Wende Zomnir), 116, 117, 128, 129, 131, 132, 149 (top), 150 (top), 151 courtesy of Scott Nathan; p. 114 (photo of Christina Bartolucci), 138 courtesy of Michelle Laurita; p. 118, 119 courtesy of Christine Gatti; pp. 114 (photo of Lisa Price), 123, 124, 125, 133, 134 courtesy of Nick Barratta; p. 127 (both) courtesy of Emile Valentine; p. 130 courtesy of Steven Kahn; p. 143 courtesy of Vincent Longo; pp. 149 (bottom), 150 (right) courtesy of Ole Henriksen; p.155 (bottom) © iStockphoto/asterix0597; p. 160 (bottom) courtesy of Paul Bricknell/Getty Images; p. 161 courtesy of Michael Rosenfeld/Getty Images.